The Key to Health

Books by The Author

Tai Chi Chuan & The Code of Life: Dragon Door Publishers St Paul USA 2000

Time For a Change: Taoist Group Publishers Essex 2002

THE KEY TO HEALTH

With Cures from East to West

GRAHAM HORWOOD

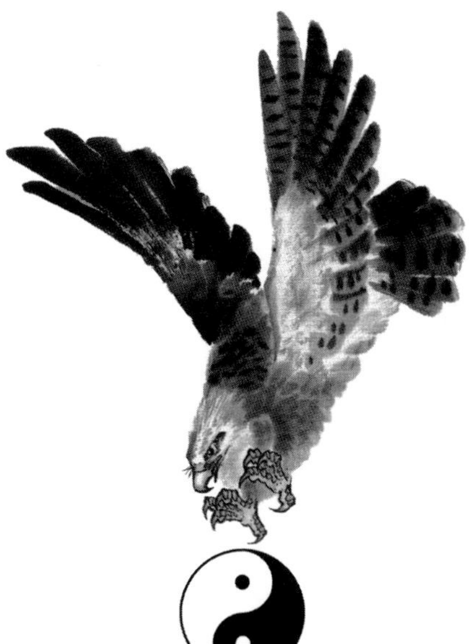

Taoist Group Publishers

Catalogue Information

Graham Horwood
Key to Health With Cures from East to West

ISBN 0-9544123-0-3

Published by The Taoist Group
66 St Andrews Road, Shoeburyness
Essex. SS3 9JJ UK 2005

Illustrations and photography by Graham Horwood.
Design by David Roskilly.

WWW.TAICHI-HORWOOD.COM

Printed and bound in Great Britain by Biddles Ltd, King's Lynn

Contents

This book is dedicated to all those who have and will strive for balance in the past, present and future. With special thanks to all who have helped me in this endeavour by either teaching, listening or applying this Universal principle and of course all the past Masters of these crafts.

PART ONE

A Balanced Diet for All Seasons and Occasions

The Principles Relating to Diet

The Natural Diet for Health

The main stay of health is to eat a balanced diet, but which one? There are a plethora of suggested diets peddled in all the media sources, books, television and also from clinicians, always changing and different. Whereas adopting the yin yang method transcends all prejudices by balancing the intake of food and its potential. Modern society and travel mean that we have lost or discarded many of our traditional diets built up by trial and error over the centuries. A simple yet effective method is to apply the yin yang principles. Knowledge of which replaces habitual eating with informed choice. Adjusting proportions and varieties of food to suit one's own constitution depending on environment, age, sex and so forth.

Yin and Yang

A self evident, but overlooked gastric mechanism, of how to judge a balanced diet, is the first place digestion takes place, being the mouth. Here there is a classic example of the interplay of yin represented by the thirty two teeth. Traditional Chinese Medicine designates these as being formed and influenced by the yin chi of the mother, as yin horizontal bone is created by the lateral forming, yin energy. (*Refer* to Part 3 on Chi Kung). This is offset by the thirty two vertebrae of the spine which are vertically determined by the yang chi of the father. The sum of which is yet another example of the 'magic' number of sixty four. This also appears as the core number of hexagrams in the I Ching. Equalled by the sixty four possible combinations or 'words' of DNA. These 'words' are needed to synthesise the twenty two or so amino acids which form the building blocks of protein for the body. (*Refer* to my book ***Tai Chi Chuan and The Code of Life.***)

Everything is beholden to the universal law of opposites and is briefly explained as follows. The world is made up of and ordered by opposite tendencies such as hot-cold, push-pull, young-old, tall-short, rich-poor neutron-electron, inner-outer and so forth which is evident but not usually recognised. These opposites happen at every level from the formation of a galaxy right down to the atom. A group of sages in ancient China, called Taoists, adopted this law of opposites into their philosophy, science and medicine. They discovered that their Universe was made of a life force which in its expanding phase was called 'yang' and when it reached its limit it changed into a contracting force, entitled 'yin'. The interacting combination of these two parts of the one force being responsible for all manifestation. This life force or chi had differing fractal levels, all obeying the law of yin and yang. Although from the same source, there was a Tao or great energy of the Universe responsible for all matter, including the planets, Earth energy and last but not least the yin yang components of the human, animal and plant kingdom. The superficial result of this unseen life force is the material world and all its variety. The Chinese character for yin indicates the dark side of a mountain with the yang being the sunny side. Thus the often misquoted and misunderstood law of yin and yang is relative to its application.

The principles of a yin or yang phase of energy can be applied to food. Therefore, if the vibrating pitch of the food is too yin or yang it will a have reciprocal effect on the DNA structure of our bodies. This is why the Genetically Modified Organisms (GMOS) are a great danger to mankind, as the balance of yin and yang have been altered artificially without the evolutionary test of time to determine the long term effects.

Therefore to stay healthy one can follow this natural law by eating natural foods which relate to the evolved array of teeth that modern humans have inherited. The twenty molars are best at chewing grains, the eight incisors are most suitable for vegetables and lastly the four canines are best suited to eat animal protein. These principles are the basis for this sensible method of balancing diet.

These yin yang principles were used successfully for millennia by Chinese scientists and doctors whose collective knowledge, from thousands of years of experience, was assembled in the sixteenth century A.D. by Li Shih-chen who compiled the *Pen-ts'ao kang-mu, The Great Pharmacopoeia.* This major work was the assimilation of centuries of diagnostic techniques, cures and remedies in fifty-two volumes. It is still revised, updated and reprinted today, currently in use being evidence of its authority and validity. The reason for this evolution of thought and experience is that China is the longest continuous civilisation.

Western Know How Versus Eastern Wisdom

A recent example of this timeless wisdom is the following case of the arrogance of power. The American Military have been seeking an antidote for malaria since the second world war. In order to protect their troops when on active duty in the tropics. Whereas a cure was uncovered in The Great Pharmacopoeia by Chinese scientists of the Institute of Malaria, Shanghai in the 1980's. The Americans knew that the Chinese had discovered this cure and put their US drive, with millions of dollars and know how into top gear to find it, but to no avail. The Chinese in the new era of Western co-operation released the formula in 1998, with the comment that the Americans had been very arrogant. Professor Ying Li who headed the Chinese team practices Tai Chi and Chi Kung everyday.

The cure is composed of substances from a wild plant, Artemesia, the daisy leaf wormwood which is ironically found along river banks all over the world, including the Potomac river in Washington. I bought a Chinese medical manual in 1976 which tells of many cures for malaria including the illusive Ch'ing Kao or Artemesia.

Unfortunately, nowadays one has to be very cautious about using herbs from China or the Far East due to the careless industrial practises since the 1940's. A lot of the herbs are contaminated by pollution and some unscrupulous suppliers even add drugs to them. So even though the recipes are accurate in appearance, the contaminating contents can be counter productive and even dangerous.

Macrobiotics

The principles of Li Shen-chen's opus were adopted by Sakurazawa Nyoichi (1893-1966), better known as George Oshawa. He formed his Shokuyo or 'macrobiotic' system, popularised by a student of his and fellow Japanese, Michio Kushi in the 1970's. Oshawa and in particular Kushi, laid out a balance of foods, with such a 'Japanese' flavour, it was impractical for a lot of people either to digest or buy the obscure expensive foods which he recommended to the West. Nevertheless George Oshawa, was cured of TB and other diseases in 1908, with these yin yang principles. He was taught by the Shinto influenced Dr Sagen Ishizuka with this traditional way of healing and balancing diet, which landed in Japan from China over the centuries. Oshawa then decided to study and practice these methods which he did successfully for fifty years. Shintoism is a Japanese hybrid of Taoism and Buddhism which has the yin yang principle at its core.

Another extraordinary example of this practical science in the frightening world of modern warfare is when Oshawa ran a health a clinic near Nagasaki. This was at the time of the atomic bombing of the City in 1945 at the end of WWII. None of his patients, although recovering from other illnesses were adversely affected by the nuclear fallout. Even though many poor Japanese living further a field than his clinic, were violently ill or killed as result of the nuclear fallout.

When the body is balanced it can fight off unwanted threats more effectively. Nuclear fall out is extremely yin, so if the protective energy of the body is kept full and yang, the yin radiation will not be absorbed. A balance diet will help keep yang protective energy clear and strong.

Chinese doctors have been applying yin yang in remedies, successfully for five thousand years, harmonising the internal energy of the body with diet, herbs and exercise. It is my intention to explain how to adopt this yin yang theme for everyday use, with everyday foods. I have been teaching, healing and practicing these methods successfully, since 1968 without resorting to any exotic formulas.

First and foremost one must bear in mind that yin and yang are relative. For example meat is more yang in comparison to the yin state of a carrot. However a carrot is more yang in relation to the very yin tomato. Although a male is generally more yang than a woman, a female can be more yang than a man. Initially it can be a bit confusing, but with a little effort it is easily comprehended. This understanding will pave the way to a practical and comprehensive way of choosing the most appropriate food for any environment or occasion. The yin yang law is relative and can be applied to any environment, climate and season.

Yin and Yang in People

The physique of a person differs depending on age, sex, build, hereditary factors, environment and of course diet. Allowing for the aforementioned criteria, a person who has a yin constitution will have one or a selection of the ensuing characteristics, albeit in varying proportions:- quiet, lethargic, thinner, fair skinned with light hair, lighter colour eyes, higher pitched voice, nose that points down, teeth that point out, wide apart eyes sometimes with the whites showing underneath, knock knees, feet that splay out, gain weight in the lower parts; the more of these, the more yin and so forth.

Whereas a more yang constitution will have a tendency to be more outgoing and lively, stocky build, thick hair, dark eyes, close set eyes, deep voice, teeth that turn in, turned up nose, tendency to have pigeon toes, bowed legs, body hair, liable to put on weight in the upper part of the body.

The relative proportion of these outward physical attributes will determine the general trend of a person. For example a thin blonde girl, with fine hair and a high voice being yin could be attracted to a thick set man with a dark complexion, curly hair and a deep voice, being more yang.

Thus a person with a yin constitution should eat more yang foods whereas a more yang individual should eat relatively more yin and so forth. One can practice this by categorising friends and family into yin and yang groupings, seeing how heredity, diet and environment effect the characteristics and constitution of the persons concerned. After a while this process will become automatic which will increase the understanding of this natural law to the benefit of all.

The following brief list of foods are arranged in a yang to yin order. Below that there is a random table of opposites.

To recap, yang is an expansive force that causes contraction, whereas yin is a contracting energy that gives rise to its opposite condition of expansion. An example of this is that salt, being a very yang substance can contract ice, which is very yin and expanded, back into a liquid. Salt is renowned as well for its properties to close open wounds also preventing infection for the same yang reason.

A Brief List of Relative Foodstuffs:

YANG	**YIN**
Wild Game	Red Meat (Farm Reared)
Red Meat	Red Fish (Bloody Fish -Tuna- Salmon etc.)
Red Fish	White Meat (Fowl etc.)/ Shell Fish.
Shell Fish/White Meat	White Fish (Plaice etc.)
White Fish	Grains
Grains	Pulses
Pulses	Root Vegetables
Root Vegetables	Leafy Green Vegetables
Leafy Green Vegetables	Herbs
Herbs	Herb Tea
Herb Tea	Regular Tea
Regular Tea	Coffee
Beer	Wine
Wine	Whisky
Whisky	Brandy

A Brief List of Yin Yang items in an unrelated order:

YANG	YIN
Salt	Sugar
Dry	Wet
Heaven	Earth
Centripetal	Centrifugal
Sun	Moon
Hot	Cold
Male	Female
Conscious	Unconscious
Fast	Slow
Outer	Inner
Day	Night
Extravert	Introvert
Sunny Side of a Mountain	Shady Aspect of a Mountain
Time	Space
Clockwise	Anti-clockwise
Light	Dark/Heavy
Expanding Force	Contracting Force
Contracted	Dilated
Activity	Passivity
Hard	Soft
Infra-red	Ultraviolet
Convex	Concave
Square	Round
Odd numbers	Even numbers
Matter	Spirit
Summer	Winter
Spring	Autumn

Yin and Yang, Einstein and Health

The West has uncovered these opposites in differing ways with such great thinkers as Einstein discovering that all matter vibrates, including the mind and body. All matter being the result of the push and pull of the interrelating atomic forces. Food also vibrates which can simply, yet effectively, be judged by its yin or yang pitch of energy. Therefore it must follow that if one eats a lot of yin vibrating food the body will absorb too much yin energy. This will cause the body to vibrate at a more yin level giving rise to a yin sickness or 'dis-ease'. An easy way to maintain or return to health is to harmonise the yin and yang of foodstuffs as well as in one's general lifestyle.

The body is comprised of yin and yang energy channels used in acupuncture etc. that are linked to the various yin and yang viscera which are disturbed by an unbalanced input of various comestibles and hectic living. So food not only sustains life but is also a medicine and a controller of health. Salt which is very yang has a yangising or contracting effect on blood vessels and organs, in particular the kidneys causing high blood pressure if taken to excess.

The word 'heal' is derived from the English word 'whole'. Therefore to be healed one must become whole, or in other words balanced. A medicine, whether it is natural or synthetic is a substance which will adjust the balance of yin and yang latency of the body's chemistry. In the West this is viewed from a chemical point of view as opposed to the energetic effects. Food also has a chemical or energetic consequence.

The average person can eat several pounds of food and many litres of fluid daily, each of which is either yin or yang, thereby having a relative outcome, even though medicine is usually more concentrated.

A person suffering from general aches and pains or in particular rheumatism will find damp or yin weather and environments, exacerbate their complaints, giving rise to more pain. Whereas in dry or hot yang climates these aches can disappear completely. Therefore if one eats more yin food the complaint will worsen but if a balanced diet is eaten one can cure the complaint or disease. (*See* Section on Joint Troubles).

An everyday, but very essential example of the interplay of yin and yang between the body and nature can be seen by the humble, yet necessary yin leafy greens and bronchial shaped vegetables like cauliflower and broccoli which increase the absorption of O_2 yin (-) by the yin organ of the lungs, supplied freely, by its natural counterpart, of the yang tree (+) which transforms the yang CO_2 back into O_2 and so forth. *(fig.1)*.

Today the first world has an enormous and exotic choice of eating but there is an ironic twist for this new found freedom. The advent of technology and the global variety of food has lead to unsustainable food production. It has become invariably tasteless requiring exotic sauces or spices to cover up the blandness. The food is also far less nutritious besides being harmful.

The method in this book is a way to balance foods with an informed choice making the individual really free. One has to decide whether it is better to invest in a wholesome diet or risk the consequences. In my opinion it is more sensible to enjoy natural food that is pleasantly prepared, knowing that it could never harm one.

Yin and Yang and The Environment

The first place to see the effects of yin and yang on eating, on a global scale, is the distribution of food from its natural habitat. The cold zones of the north and south poles are extreme yin, whilst the hot equator is full yang. Applying the law of opposites, food consumed in cold climates should be more yang, whereas at the equator more yin, to compensate for the climatic energy differential. Take the case of spices which grow naturally in hot climates, although hot to the tongue are actually, a yin food as they cause the blood to thin, thereby

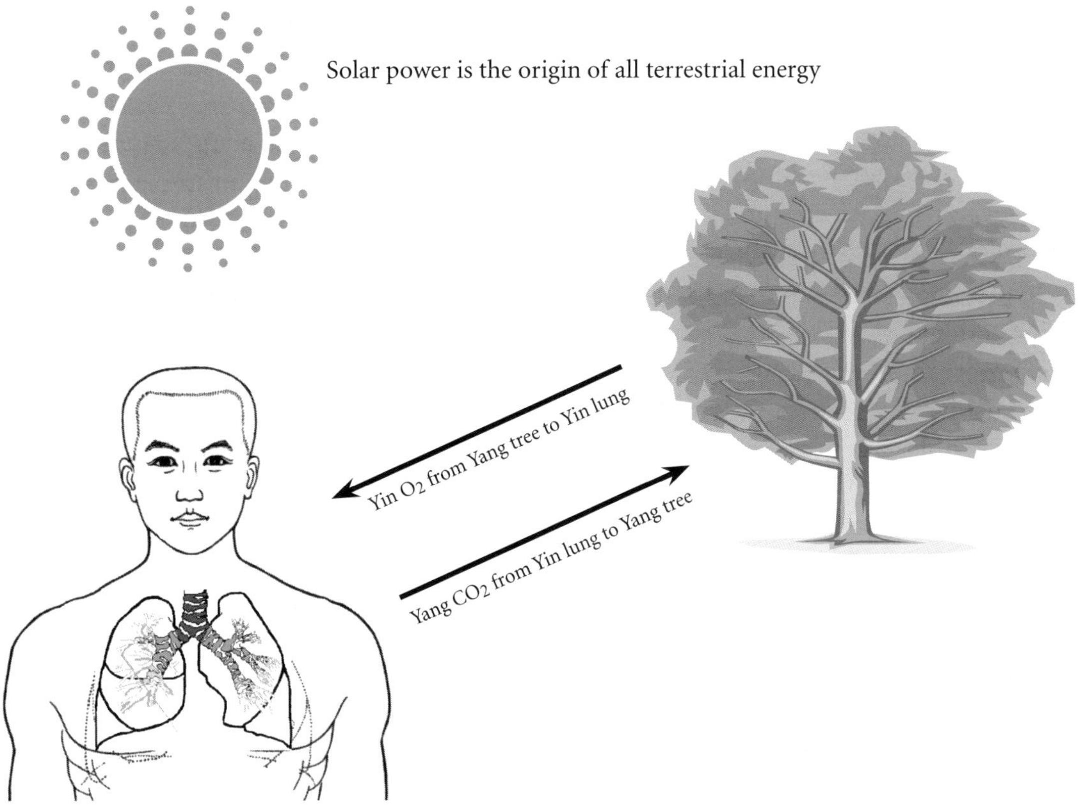

Figure 1: The lung is a yin organ, being like an inverted tree accepting the vital O_2 and post birth essence of the Sun. The body expels the yang CO_2 which is food for, and processed by nature. This is a classic case of the harmonious law of opposites in action, rarely appreciated, now often abused.

'yinnising' the metabolism to keep the body cooler.

So, if one overeats yin food in the northern hemisphere, it will cause the body to cool unnaturally. The exception is high altitudes, being very yang, where spices are used to thin the blood for O_2 transportation. It is unfortunate for peoples who have migrated from the tropics to cooler zones with their familiar equatorial spicy diets with exotic ingredients. This speedy migration did not take into consideration the climate differences often causing mysterious clusters of illnesses amongst minority cultures in their new adopted lands.

The organism will always try to redress the balance naturally. This automatic mechanism is achieved by draining away the reserves of internal energy. When the internal energy is exhausted by overworking to balance the excesses of yin and yang, the body's defences break down resulting in disease.

Vitamins, Pollution and GMO's

Another classic misconception of preserving health is the quick fix myth of synthesised vitamins and minerals which will aid the organism initially but have less and less effect over time as the body needs these substances from their natural sources to be assimilated properly. The so called healthy option of Vitamin C from imported oranges, grapefruits and lemons out of season and climate will produce counter effects. Citrus fruits are very yin which again cool the body down unnaturally in colder climates. One symptom gives rise to cold hands and feet which shows that the organism is becoming too yin thus reducing the resistance to the cold and colds. This can lead to rheumatism, arthritis and chest problems such as bronchitis and asthma. All of which are triggered by the excess yin of the citrus fruits even though they contain an essential vitamin. Vitamin C should be sourced from indigenous fruit and vegetables in season.

An important factor determining health is the habitual environment where one lives or works. Where the same yin yang rules apply. Places to avoid are the dangerous man-made, micro-climates found near power lines, antennas, radio masts etc.. All of these give off strong electromagnetic currents which yinnise the body. All electro-smogs due to their extreme yin inducing qualities, yinnise the body primarily reducing the immune function. Equally the home should be free of synthetic fibres and building materials whenever possible as well as the electro-magnetic fields created by electrical equipment. So avoid long term exposure to TV's, computers, clock radios near beds, hairdriers, microwave ovens, radio antennas, mobile phones and so forth.

Leukaemia (-) clusters are found near nuclear plants (-), high energy cables (-) and so forth. It is an extreme yin (-) effect on the bone marrow where healthy blood cells are produced. The yin white blood cells (-) become abundant or of poor quality. Whereas the yang (+) blood cells and platelets are reduced.

Leukaemia symptoms are flu like having many yin characteristics including:- tiredness, weight loss, difficulty in breathing, loss of appetite, abdominal discomfort and bruising. Infection, bone pain, and anaemia are also symptoms with haemorrhaging also occurring in areas such as the gums and the nose.

The most dangerous unseen yin danger is nuclear radiation, Chernobyl being the most recent terrifying example of the long term and drastic effects of this type of unnecessary method of power production. Nuclear power has more to do with the nuclear arms race than energy supply. The main cause of the many premature deaths in and around Chernobyl, is leukaemia.

Therefore if the diet is not balanced it will reduce our ability to cope with unfriendly environmental conditions, stress and pathogens.

Here I have compiled a yin yang diet to return or sustain health, as well as acting as a learning tool on how to incorporate and enjoy one's own preferences in a balanced way. After appreciating the subtleties of balancing the internal potential of food, it can be modified to suit individual tastes and customs. However if one falls ill, no matter how serious, one can adhere strictly to this health guide, permitting the internal energy of the body to stabilise thus enhancing its ability to fight back against the illness, besides acting as wholesome nutrition.

There are so many different ways of cooking food I suggest, at the outset, to prepare organic food in the traditional manner but adjusting the proportions as laid out below. However avoid cooking in non-stick and aluminium pans both of which are poisonous. Ideally use stainless steel and or fired clay cooking vessels and their like.

The following balance of food is geared for a general modern lifestyle for a temperate climate with four seasons, like the United Kingdom. The balance of ingredients should be adjusted depending on climate, season and physical exertion (sport/pregnancy etc.). When applying this method for different conditions, food should be generally more yang in cooler seasons and cooked for longer, in ovens and closed pots. In hotter periods and climates, the nutriments should be lightly cooked or eaten raw, increasing yin types of foods.

Industrialised Food

On a final and seriously dangerous note, I wish to issue a grave warning about the quality of food. One must always try to buy and eat fresh food, free of preservatives and additives, which have been grown organically and prepared as naturally as possible. The so-called approved additives and agri-cides have never been tested by any Western government agency as a collective cocktail or over a long period. There are many unacceptable claims from the scientific community concerning the so-called safe substances. This is highly dubious science when this has only been tested in laboratories not in society for an extended period. The reason for the lack of safe testing is purely economics. These noxious substances have only been tested separately on innocent animals, for inconclusive periods of time by the companies who profit from the sale and production of these chemicals.

Irradiation of foods is another unseen trick of the food industry of prolonging the ever-desired shelf life, particularly of 'fresh' foods. It is declared by many large food chains that they will advise if foods have been irradiated. This is as difficult to police as detecting GMOS. Also it is not legally apparent how these should be labelled. For example what if the food was irradiated outside the European Union or at sea without prior knowledge of the purchaser. It is an unseen process needing sophisticated equipment to detect. It is increasingly more and more difficult to rely on the good intention, alone, of any large enterprise. A rough way to judge this, is to see if fresh food lasts unnaturally long and stays looking 'fresh' without going off such as salads, vegetables and sea foods. If the food does not decay naturally, it is likely that it has been blasted with radiation.

Radiation 'preserves' food by making it more yin. This unacceptable synthetic yinising slows things down, preventing decay, but dangerously. Whereas chilling and freezing do not. In the case of radiation the yin is pernicious with its invisible effects being passed on to the consumer in turn 'slowing' down the body's processes unnaturally. Other preserved foods including the chilled varieties are quickly and easily yangised by heat which is certainly not the case for irradiated foods.

Another proof of unsustainable food production which is not only poisoning the land but the consumer as well is where farm workers have to be dressed in protective clothing. These unfortunate workers resemble space travellers whilst applying these 'safe' substances to our comestibles. In many cases they are legally obliged to wear protective apparel, face masks and so forth, whilst spreading these 'harmless' products on the land and animals.

The old chestnut that these agro-chemicals and industrialised food production are simply to provide increased bounty for the sake of humanity is a lie. It is a spurious argument of corporate self deception and self justification, being in denial in order to cover up the exclusive profit driven motives to control food production. As always the people who pay are the innocent consumer, not only with their pockets, but also with their health.

Organic farming has been proved by many farmers around the world to be safer and in the long term more economical than modern intensive farming. The result of irresponsible industrial farming is becoming more and more evident as the long term effects of these toxic cocktails manifest themselves in humans as the increase of allergies, bizarre new illnesses, cancers, immune and neurological disorders, loss of fertility in both men and women and so forth. The incidences of children born without eyes is twice as prevalent in the country as metropolitan districts, as is the increase of asthma in rural areas, to name but a few out of town dilemmas.

Wraps, smells and floors

In 2004 research found that over three generations of families, the grandchildren had absorbed the highest levels of chemicals such as - polychlorinated and polybrominated biphenyls and ethers used in insulation, coolants, flame retardants, textiles, plastics, clothing and furniture proven to cause liver cancer and brain cell detonation. Also there are the phthalates developed for Clingfilm, pvc flooring, shampoos and skin lotion, children's toys and perfume causing kidney damage and asthma. Then there are the smells made by artificial 'musks' added to most perfume, aftershave, soap, air freshener, cleaning products and detergents linked to miscarriages and liver damage. Certain chemicals in anti- perspirants, like aluminium, have been discovered in cancerous breast tissue. Perfluorinated chemicals are used in fast food containers, non-stick pans, carpets and furniture as stain protectors, the health risks of these are bladder cancer. Last but not least are the volatile organic compounds (VOC's) that are found in most types of aerosol sprays, being equally as toxic for the organism, which are to be avoided.

Frankenstein Foods

God only knows what Genetically Modified Organisms will do; certainly these GMO's have not been produced for the benefit of the consumer. These Frankenstein foods are produced by corporate monsters in homage to the new god of greed and power. I predict more disasters emanating from this immature and untested formula for improving balance sheets, by the unnecessary manipulation of plant and animal DNA. At the moment the paying public are being used as cheap experiments.

To sum up if any substance or deed is carried out without the true well-being of the recipient in mind, the dark malevolence of the act or substance will always have a destructive effect. History is the proof of this. This view was echoed on the UK's BBC Television, in 1998, by a professor from Cornell University, Ithaca, N.Y., USA. He pointed out that the Organo-phosphates (agro-chemicals) which are widely used as pesticides throughout the world, were astonishingly developed at the chemical factory where the inmates worked, at Auschwitz during World War II. The Organo-phosphate compounds were fed into the gas chambers of this infamous death camp, in order to speed up the Nazi plan of mass genocide. Sarin, an Organo-phosphate is a nerve gas stockpiled by many countries being an efficient weapon of mass destruction. Sarin was employed in the terrorist attack on a Tokyo subway train, killing many people in March 1995.

Hopefully more and more people will become conscious of these facts and demanding the return of natural foods. This will improve and fortify one's health, helping to fend off any hidden undesirable elements from food and the environment. Last but not least it will help to protect the environment by supporting careful and sustainable food production besides thwarting the heinous processes of corporate self-interest economics.

General Guide for a Balanced Diet Applying The Principles of Yin and Yang

The following is best suited to an environment that has four distinct seasons. The balance of food can be adjusted to allow for variations in climate. More hot more yin, more cold more yang etc..

All food whenever possible should be carefully selected from organic and free range sources that sustain the environment, people and animals.

Yang Foods

1) Each meal should consist mainly of food from fresh natural plant origin, 50% of which is organic whole cereal grains such as brown rice, whole wheat and its by products i.e. bread, whole wheat chapatis, whole wheat noodles and pasta, barley, millet, rye, rye bread, oats, oatmeal, cous-cous, corn, corn on the cob, buckwheat pancakes. Including the occasional top up with preferred animal or seafood from safe sustainable sources, such as fresh fish, free range poultry and wild game. Preferably avoiding completely or if desired the occasional moderate consumption of organic red meat such as beef, pork, lamb or their by-products. Increased physical activity requires more yang food, preferably carbohydrate supported by some seafood or animal protein if desired. Dairy foods although yang and widely consumed in Western societies are acidic and a body 'clogger' so best avoided if possible. Dairy food was originally a way to conserve protein in cold climates. This is less relevant today with central heating, modern houses and travel. Occasional eating of organic dairy products will do no great harm. Just remember Bovine Spongiform Encephalopathy (BSE) et al. will be in the food chain for years despite the claims to the contrary from the vested interests.

Yin Foods

2) 20-30% organic vegetables in season, the more yang, root variety for winter and more leafy, yin in summer including fresh salads. This can include seaweed which is becoming more popular having a natural high mineral content. Be careful of its origin due to sea pollution.

3) 10-15% beans, pulses i.e. chick and split peas, lentils, black eye beans, kidney beans, as part of the main meal which can be cooked in stews or in soups etc..

4) 5% nuts, seeds and seasonal fruits eaten with care will add protein and variety to diet but prevent habitual intake of exotic and tropical foods like oranges, kiwis, mangoes, bananas etc. which 'yinnise' the body. Conventional confection e.g. sweets, chocolate, biscuits, cakes should be moderate due to the high sugar content, colouring, additives and animal by-products such as gelatine, GMO soya lecithin, etc..

Liquids

5) A sensible intake of 'clean' uncomplicated fluids will not overly effect the yin/yang balance

of the diet. Liquid is quickly dealt with by a normal metabolism. Therefore depending on activity, sweat ratio etc. one should drink around ½-1 litre or so a day depending on liquid discharge and activity. Try to avoid drinking 'tap' water, unless properly filtered as it contains a chemical cocktail of agro-chemicals such as the Organo-phosphates, fertilisers, heavy metals, chlorine, bacteria, phenols (the gender benders) and fluoride which is considered carcinogenic and banned in certain discerning countries.

Soft drinks are not soft but very hard. Hard on the body, regular cokes, colas and the so called tropical drinks etc. are a cocktail of chemicals and sugar which besides damaging teeth, will stress liver and kidney function. Reliable scientific studies in the United States have linked sugar free foods and diet drinks containing aspartame to premature Alzheimer's disease also giving rise to severe, sometimes irreversible, symptoms of Multiple Sclerosis. I doubt if it is worth the risk for anybody to indulge in these toxins. Even worse is the expensive advertising of these substances targeted at the young and innocent. The can and its design logo cost much more to produce than the toxic liquid it contains.

Regular tea (commercial Indian etc.) and coffee contain natural stimulants like caffeine and tannin etc.. These are highly processed containing hidden chemicals which will add to the collective cocktail but will do no great harm if drunk in moderation. Far better to be replaced with natural decaffeinated coffee and pure Indian or Chinese green tea and the usual herbal infusions available now from supermarkets in the UK. In Okinawa and parts of China green tea is linked to the low incidence of cancer amongst the population. Please note that teas are made from the leaf of a plant thus being the receptor of all sprays so always buy organic infusions.

Alcohol

Alcohol is a yin substance being the distillation and or fermentation of grain or fruit etc.. Originally alcohol was produced to alter the state of consciousness for religious rituals. This practice is probably derived from our hunter-gatherer forebears who ate over ripened berries with the resultant mind altering effects. In the Amazon there are still Indians who do this in order to heighten their inner senses for hunting purposes, with great effect. Shamans from Arctic Lapland achieve the same results with certain fungi in order to track reindeer and hunt wild game. Alcohol like all mind altering substances lowers the veil of consciousness allowing access to the unconscious which is a time space void, letting one see round corners. This intuitive ability to 'see' in the unconscious can be natural function in some people; (*Refer to* the Stress Section in this book). However like all synthetic practices if overindulged will lose its poignancy. This property is now used as a modern 'anaesthetic' which yinnises the brain giving a very temporary relief from the pressures and stresses of modern life. It is generally abused but if understood in relation to yin and yang and diet it can be a method of controlled relaxation for some. It is a yin substance that burdens liver function, the more the degrees of alcohol, the more yin it is. An excess will always cause distress. The more yang alcohols are the grain based ones such as beer and whisky. The more yin being wine and brandy and so forth.

If alcohol is drunk in moderation and not misused, it will do no great harm. Again one has to do some homework and be selective on the type and quantity of the ingredients in the preparation of alcoholic beverages. The highly profitable drinks industry is not interested in health but its balance sheet. One of the major costs of a product is the slick advertising of these mass produced substances. They have long shelf lives assured by the content of a great deal of additives to preserve this highly lucrative stance. So be selective, seeking out naturally produced products which are available and can also support local or cottage industries concerned with ecology. GMOS are now used in the production of alcohol which are unlabelled.

Taboo Foods

Some popular foods to be avoided whenever possible or eaten in moderation are :- tomatoes, potatoes, aubergines, egg plant, avocados, yams, asparagus, spinach, beets, bananas, all being very yin for northern climates. Potatoes and tomatoes are related to the same plant family as Deadly Nightshade also containing oxalic acid which burdens the liver and can leach iron out of the blood.

Sugar, White Death

Since the heinous birth of this massive consumer market based on the slave trade, to its present day corporate exploitation, the sugar trade has been shrouded in darkness.

Therefore avoid refined sugar whenever possible, but also be aware that all sugar, raw cane, organic or otherwise, is extremely yin. Excess intake will cause the body to become yin, causing tiredness, listlessness and lethargy initially, before the body becomes more addicted and ill.

Ensure you always read the label carefully in order to correctly ascertain the contents and amounts of sugar in the food product. Also be aware of the 'hidden' sugar content labelling, e.g. sucrose etc..

Sugar is a very profitable way for the food industry, to bulk out food cheaply as well as being a pernicious way to preserve shelf life and increase profits. Large amounts of sugar are to be found in many foodstuffs where the quantity is unspecified; including soft drinks, alcohol, cakes, biscuits, bread, sauces, ready cook meals, ice-cream, desserts, confection, chocolate and jams etc.. Sometimes over half the product or more can contain this cheap and dangerous, yet addictive substance.

Regular sugar consumption, whether hidden in drinks, foods or used as a sweetener will cause tooth decay, as well as reducing liver and kidney function, thus weakening joints, tendons and muscles.

Sugar attacks the immune function as well as being a major cause of diabetes. All sugars are extremely yin and make the mind and body excessively yin, especially the refined sugars. Sugar is a poor carbohydrate that forms into a yin acidic substance in the body, besides being difficult to digest and purge from the system, it is addictive. Hence its usage by the food industry. It used to be sold as a high energy body food, but in effect it actually slows down the mind and body acting as a sort of anaesthetic, after a short lived high.

George Oshawa considered that a major factor in the onset of leprosy can be caused by refined sugar consumption, hence he called it white death during his time as a healing missionary in Africa!

Sugar binges are commonly used to forget or to be 'spoilt' as a treat, acting as a compensation for a hurt or loss. In Complementary Medicine this can be allied to the fact that mother's milk is naturally sweet. Even if experienced or not, this ambrosia is in the collective memory bank of DNA. Therefore this human nectar is akin to the unconditional kindness of an adoring mother as she selflessly feeds her helpless, yet nurtured offspring.

Cooking

7) Always cook foodstuffs or prepare salads, sparingly, with unrefined virgin pressed culinary oils of natural origin such as cold pressed virgin sesame, corn, olive oil, sunflower and safflower oils. Oils are yin substances so use with care.

Seasoning

8) Lightly season foods, if necessary, with unrefined sea salt from an unpolluted source, in moderation. Salt was a sign of wealth in the past hence the word 'salary, so there is a misguided tradition that salty food is a sign of wealth. It must be used very carefully as it yangises the system. One dangerous effect being high blood pressure as the kidneys are yangised or contracted unnaturally thus reducing their function as well as restricting the flow of blood in yangised arteries, putting the heart under unnecessary duress. A simple test to see if there is too much salt in one's food is that it should not taste salty. A very acceptable savoury substitute which contains pound for pound more calcium than cheese or milk is 'sesame salt'. This is made from 1 part unrefined sea salt to 10 parts of organic sesame seeds which are lightly roasted together, then ground to taste. Sesame salt or gomasio can be used to ease an asthma attack. (*See* Asthma Section). Also there are natural soya sauces available from most health food shops. Commercial soya sauce is normally a chemical cocktail to be avoided at all costs.

Garlic is a wonderful seasoning besides which, will strengthen the immune system, but it is a yin substance so too much will have a counter effect. About a clove a day is more than ample to season and protect. It can be given to animals as well to keep down infection.

9) Cook food with as little waste as possible, keeping cooking times to a minimum, always considering that the nutritional value is as important as flavour.

GMOS

10) Last but not least, please check all the labels so as to avoid industrialised foods and artificial additives, colouring and preservatives including sugar, and GMOS. All being unacceptable extremes of yin and yang which drain the intrinsic energy of the individual. Many substances sold as safe in the UK are banned in the US or Europe. These unwanted additives are added to increase shelf life and profitability and not designed to improve health. Unnatural food will damage the internal organs, especially the heart, lungs, kidneys, pancreas, intestines and liver.

Overview

This health guide, once understood, will reap great rewards. It can be modified with a little thought, to suit one's own cultural, religious and environmental criteria by adapting and adopting the yin yang concept of balancing fresh wholesome food to taste, season and latitude.

When one becomes ill, eat and drink simply, reducing all the heavy foods especially the extremes, adhering to a vegetarian diet of 70% yang to 30 % yin foods, until well.

To conclude, one should eat foods that are local and in season which for the UK being still a temperate zone. The diet should generally contain 70% yang food to 30% yin. Always choose foods from natural organic sources comprising of (50%) grains plus some fish or animal protein, (20%) pulses, balanced by (30%) yin foods, preferably vegetables and limited amounts of seasonal fruit. One can adjust the amounts depending on the climate, i.e. so if the weather is very yang, then more yin food can be eaten and vice versa.

Freedom and Travel

With practice and perseverance the yin yang principles will become second nature not only in choosing food but also lifestyle, allowing one to judge the most acceptable balanced way of living, wherever one ends up. This rare, yet available freedom if persevered with, will save lots of potential trouble. Cancer and many other illnesses are on the increase. Twenty five years ago one in forty were destined to have a cancer, now it is deemed to strike one in three in the first world.

Excesses of yin and yang tend to be forcibly redressed on the metabolism by climate change which can manifest itself with loose bowels, fevers and so forth, so if one voyages to a distant land try and find out the local foodstuffs and their type of preparation adjusting one's food a few days before travel to assist the changeover and avoid spoiling a holiday or business trip with a 'Delhi Belly' syndrome.

Otherwise the body can react with upset stomachs, colds, coughs and flu as it throws off the excess yin or yang from the previous climate or environment.

Normal healthy people can wander from the above yin/yang concepts using common sense and care. The body is flexible enough to cope with small changes without any danger. The symptoms of the common cold are often simulated when the body is expelling toxins. But any stress on the body's natural reserves will use more of the vital energy or essential 'chi' which is finite. This ability to recover wanes as the essential 'chi' is diminished naturally by age or persistent illness. (*See* Chi Kung in Part 3).

Whenever convenient, try and avoid late eating, preferably for at least three hours before retiring. Food consumed late at night is not fully digested and can lead to the body storing the undigested food as fat or mucous. The nutritious value of food is digested more effectively when yang chi is waxing from early morning up to midday. The body's digestive ability diminishes accordingly from midday to midnight, as chi wanes proportionately from yang to yin. One can use daylight to assess the scale of yang to yin energy. Dusk and dawn being a transition of one to the other.

There are other determining factors which must be considered and harmonised to ensure health besides diet including stress and environment including habitat. A mountain is a yang region whereas the coast is more yin. The town or city is more yin than the countryside being more yang. The tropics are more yang and the temperate zones more yin and so forth. Also pollution plays a great factor which is usually very yin such as factory and incinerator emissions. There are also inherited factors including genetics, pathogens and harmful bacteria. Last but not least is a disturbed psyche which will give rise one way or another to all the above. A personal trauma can induce many illnesses from the common cold to cancer, thus reducing the immune function. An old adage is he/she has lost the will to live due to the loss of a loved one etc.. This is covered in more detail on how the psyche interferes with the organism in ***Tai Chi Chuan & The Code of Life*** and in more detail in my book ***Time for a Change.***

Tai Chi and Cancer

In 2006 a male student, 50 years old, informed me of a doctor's diagnosis of throat cancer. He had been a long time smoker and had a haphazard 'organic' diet as well as doing Tai Chi. He first came to me in 1997 for some for aches and pains. I dealt with the kidney and liver chi deficiency, advising a wholesome diet, with appropriate exercise, and as ever I stressed the importance of taking notice of the inner aspects of the psyche by way of dreams because they are a dialogue with the unconscious which has amazing and fascinating potential.

I asked him for dream material, whereupon he told me that he did not take notice or remember many, but with effort recounted a long term recurrent nightmare of choking on various objects which with association related to negative experiences concerning his childhood, family including his step mother. I suggested that he should continue the dream work, but unfortunately he declined.

When I showed him the dream material notes that he gave me back in 1997, he was visibly moved, seeing the connection. I recommended a strict organic brown rice diet (*See* diet section) to 'starve' the cancer and visualisation techniques from Chi Kung which are also used in modern day China as in the Shanghai Sanatorium of Chi Kung*.

For example find a quiet, natural spot preferably facing the early morning sun and breathe in pure, clean white chi from the sun to the tan tien in order to build up a store of 'fresh' chi (*See* Chi Kung section). Then imagine drawing in the pure, white healing chi from the sun to the place of discomfort or at issue then visualise exhaling away, the dark, turbid chi from the effected area. This will help healing as well as pain management. Do both chi kungs, in sets of four 'in and out' cycles.

Nevertheless due to a destructive anima problem, (*See* ***Collected Works CG Jung Volume 9 i & ii*** - and Von Franz - ***Puer Aeturnus***), he opted for the torment of conventional treatment, being radio and chemo therapy.

At publication he is still under doctor's orders. If he survives the treatment he can still opt for diet and chi kung to assist recovery and maintain remission. I added this experience because of a dream I had after visiting him in hospital, showing that radio and chemo therapy can be torture.

* In July 1957 The Shanghai Municipal Qigong Sanitorium was founded and The Ministry of Health of the People's Republic of China set up forums to consolidate and scientifically test the Chi Kungs from all over China that had been transmitted by Taoists and the likes of the Yang Family over the millennia. Representatives from seventeen provinces, municipalities and autonomous regions of China covering millions of people were drawn together. Thereafter scientists adopted modern

scientific instruments and methods to test the efficacy of Chi kungs from all over China especially in Beijing and Shanghai with a comprehensive and multi-disciplinary approach. Thus Chi Kung was scientifically proven to be an effective healing discipline, for promoting health and curing disease. Tai Chi Chuan is a moving Chi Kung.

Cancer, The Doctor and Yin Yang

Michio Kushi told me an interesting story of a medic who headed a clinic in the United States in the 1970's. The chief doctor went for his regular medical check up after which the results shocked him as he had contracted cancer which had spread throughout the lymph system, being incurable. The ambitious deputy head of the clinic realised that he would now become the boss with all its trappings, so he did not seem too distressed by the news he broke to his senior colleague that his life span was short.

The dying doctor decided to tidy up his affairs as well as visiting, by car, some relatives across the country. After having a break he saw a hitch hiker, his first reaction was that this layabout could be dangerous to pick up. But the dying man relented as he needed some company and had little to lose, offering the young man a lift. They got talking and the condemned driver admitted his plight. Whereupon the hitchhiker casually said he knew a clinic that cured cancers by diet, exercise and soul searching. He initially scoffed at such a place because he was a scientist. Then on reflection, as he had nothing to lose, he asked where it was.

The holistic centre was run by Michio Kushi in Boston. Intrigued he detoured to this apparent magical centre for healing, as it was in his general direction. After some effort and a change in mind set, he was cured using the criteria of balancing the yin and yang in his diet and his soul.

He returned to his old clinic and got himself re-tested and the cure was confirmed much to the surprise of his old medical team.

I recommend a book ***The Cancer Prevention Diet*** by Michio Kushi and Alex Jack. (*See also the **Key to Health** section at www.taichi-horwood.com*)

Jaws' Cure

During the more liberal 1980's in the UK there were more open television documentaries on all subjects including health as well as politics. During a BBC Horizon broadcast on cancer a therapist from the east coast of the USA, had encouraged a cancer patient to imagine the most feared thing eating away his cancer. The Floridian concerned cited a great white shark which he visualised gnawing away his tumour. He recovered and at the time of the film he showed the camera a large tooth from a great white which he wore around his neck as a souvenir.

Please remember the psyche and Jung's aphorism - *'The body is the mere visibility of the soul and the soul is the psychological experience of the body.'*

Yin and Yang and The Soul

All illness is allied to a sickness in the soul. This is the main reason for the plethora of hit and miss cures from all disciplines, natural or mainstream. If the soul of a person is not at rest, it will manifest itself as fate regardless of any attempted remedy. The best way to adjust this factor is to turn inward to the inner truth which is available and free to all every night, in dreams.

If one wants to discover why the soul has manifested an illness, simply look at the symptoms and see what they are telling you. For example if one's right leg is hurting, it could be one does not want to advance in life. Asthma could be a burden 'sitting' on the chest. Cancer is something added to the body. Jung speculated that it was a serious problem too awful for the individual to accept, which then 'grips' one in the body like the claws of a crab. Back trouble could be a painful experience from the past as often the back represents the past and the front the future and so forth.

Jung and Dreams

A person will tend to eat and behave in such a way as to encourage the symptoms rather as if part of the soul is saying 'you will face this, one way or the other'. One has to honestly listen and analyse the inner objective voice of dreams and outpourings of the psyche. Dream messages act as a compensation for the outer life, just as yin balances yang. This impartial medium will dig up the reason which is always there, but usually under a lot of debris. Sometimes if the person cannot face the problem directly, whilst outer healing is taking place the repressed factors arise in a quid pro quo format, sometimes causing fits of emotion or necessary depression. Depression is nature's way of cooling the ego and thus allowing the unconscious to filter its message through to consciousness. A sometimes unpleasant but useful tool of enlightenment. I must refer the reader to volume 16, *The Psychology of the Transference*, from Jung's collected works for a full dissertation on the subject of the necessary darkening of the soul on the path of wholeness.

The process of healing can be summed up, in Jung's statement: "*That the body is the mere visibility of the soul and the soul is the psychological experience of the body*".

The definition of a soul is difficult to determine as there are many interpretations of what a soul is. I shall adopt a Jungian concept of a soul being the unique part of a person which strives for wholeness. It seems that initially the soul is often inter-dependent on collective values, such as family, race, religion etc.. Jung's option to find a personal inner truth and meaning, was to individuate away from these collective associations without alienating them.

Briefly people's inner beings, by way of projection, are influenced by and intermingled with the various groups according to the level of unconscious association. Firstly there is the family group soul, comprising simply of the parents and siblings, which can spread out into the extended family which is apparent in Asian or Italian type extended family collectives.

The next collective distinction is the area of residential identity such as village, town, city or county. Then the collective identity flows out into a religious and or national soul. Lastly an important and ignored level is the Anima Mundi, the world soul which joins all mankind. This is now prevalent in the global economy. An unfortunate advocate of the Anima Mundi was Giordano Bruno who was burned at the stake as a heretic by the Inquisition for his assumptions on February 17th, 1600 in Italy. He inspired Galileo amongst many innovators.

DNA, Spirit and The Unconscious

The same rule applies to each stratum, the more collective the more unconscious. This does not mean that one should be alien to or not support any of these collectives. They form the necessary social factions which create cohesive families and societies. On the other hand, one should not be unconsciously controlled by them. Many collective 'blind' passions are produced by these clusters which can lead to the cumulative misguided responses of war mongering, racial hatred, religious prejudice and the now all too prevalent classes of self interest economic groups.

These aggregate souls could explain the cause of the seemingly unnecessary collective disasters of the innocents in famines, epidemics and so forth. Jung realised during World War Two that the collective psyche of the time was responsible for the collective atrocities of the day. This was engendered by the all too human capacity of inertia, self-deception and self-justification.

This collective phenomenon could explain the hereditary diseases and disasters that befall some families. When an innocent child for no apparent reason is born handicapped or becomes ill, this could be the result of a collective family destiny, akin to the Oriental concept of fate or retribution (karma). Whether there is a transmigration of souls or reincarnation is debatable and beyond proof. Equally there could be a sort of 'karmic' set of DNA messages which are inherited by a species, race or a family.

If one bears in mind that the DNA molecule that shapes a 'family' trait is inherited from forbears, nevertheless it is equally as possible for this memory bank of physical information to also hold psychic data. This possibility explains why twins who, separated at birth, after meeting later in life, although being brought up by different families, discover identical habits, as well as inherent features. Characteristics of human beings are definitely passed down. Easily identified by the historical family traits confirmed in all manner of families over the centuries. This is particularly evident amongst the ruling classes, due to their high profile. They also had the wherewithal to record their past with portraits and historical documents. This is highlighted by the Hapsburg lisp of the European monarchy or the Medici nose and so forth.

The public face of modern medicine is still too dogmatic at the moment to accept the existence of the soul or its sphere of influence. Thereby missing this area of study which Jung developed at the turn of the twentieth century.

Dr. Jung always maintained that the inner aspect of a person was the most significant and the outer values were mere occurrences. This is difficult to understand from the present biased, material worldview. It is neither the length nor the outside appearance of any life form that is important but the inner experience of the soul which is paramount. Always remembering that life and consciousness in themselves are precious gifts, irreverently squandered by many. Therefore the more conscious one can become, the more healing will take place on an individual or a collective basis.

Inner Voice of Healing

Here is an article from a UK broadsheet newspaper, The Independent, on Friday 19th December 1997 headed: ‘*Voices warned of* ’.

“A woman who heard voices telling her there was something wrong was later diagnosed with a brain tumour despite the scepticism of her GP. The unnamed woman had first accepted counselling and medication fearing she was going mad, but when the voices returned after she had a holiday, she went back to her doctor and demanded a brain scan. He reluctantly agreed and was criticised by colleagues for accepting what his patient’s hallucinatory voices were telling her, until the scan disclosed the tumour.

Writing in the British Medical Journal, the GP Dr Ikechukwu Azuonye describes how the woman was operated on successfully and made a full recovery. On regaining consciousness, she heard voices for the last time when she claimed they told her: ‘We are pleased to have helped you. Goodbye’.”

I will leave the last word in this part to Professor Carl Gustav Jung;

“Dream the Myth on”.

General Daily Food Guide

This general guide is for a temperate climate with four defined seasons which can be modified according to taste, personal preferences, season and climatic zone.

Teeth and Food

As stated above the teeth are evolutionary indicators of how and what we should eat. The majority of human teeth are pre-molars and molars, twenty for an adult, which are best suited to grinding grains, cereals, legumes and other seeds, with the eight incisors advocating the eating and cutting of vegetables and lastly the four canine teeth designed for tearing apart animal food.

Therefore a rule of thumb is to have a diet which follows this ratio. This works out five parts of grain type foods to two parts of vegetable matter and lastly one part animal protein, (5:2:1.). One should try and eat more before midday and less afterwards. Avoiding eating food for at least three hours before retiring. Choose fresh food that is in season which has been grown or reared naturally, i.e. organically, from the same region or climatic zone in which you live. The following suggestions are for a temperate zone with four seasons. However these are not to be followed blindly but to act as a guide. Allowing for personal preferences, always adopt the magic formula of 70% yang to 30 % yin food, of mainly plant origin. Also the quality and type of food should be adjusted according to climate and metabolism, but try to keep the variety, type and colour of food as diverse as possible.

Whenever possible, allowing for travel, work etc. try and buy fresh food that looks wholesome with little or preferably no artificial flavouring, colouring and additives. Unnatural additives i.e. chemicals, agricides, GMOS, colouring, e numbers etc. are harmful and can kill. Reduce salt and salty foods check labels as salt is hidden as a preservative to increase shelf life and profits, dairy food (due to high fat content and hormones and BSE etc.) and all refined sugar and sugar by-products used as a cheap, yet pernicious bulking additive and preservative, confection, soft drinks etc.. Eat fresh organic food whenever practical.

Breakfast:

Wholemeal toast, rice cakes, rye toasts, good quality crisp-bread with organic butter or spreads to suit taste.

Organic porridge or whole grain non-GMO cereals, with minimum quantities of organic milk and honey or unrefined sugar, to taste. (porridge being more suitable for colder weather).

Eggs mixed with fish and or rice as in kedgeree, are a good source of energy in winter, (winter sports etc.)

Fruit compôte or occasional seasonal fruit - avoid citrus fruit and drink and if desired, only in warmer weather.

Preferably herb tea especially if 'detoxing', or organic tea or coffee, with sensible amounts of milk and only use natural sweetener, like honey or unrefined sugar if needed, never artificial sweeteners, being very harmful.

Midday Meal:

Organic Pasta: spaghetti-noodles-ravioli etc. with vegetables, keep tomato and cheese to a minimum: Rice dishes (only have organic brown rice as the husk will retain all the agri-cides) like risotto of vegetables and fish and seafood: Tofu (non GMO) with mixed vegetables and rice, millet, cous cous etc. Chick pea/lentil and vegetable pasties and samosas. Buckwheat and Rye sealed pancakes with fillings of mixed vegetables: Savoury millet/ rice and vegetable balls, (ideal for packed lunches): Cous Cous and vegetables with minimal spices, avoid all spices in cold weather. Seafood and vegetables or salads in summer with wholemeal and rye type breads. If on a detox or recuperating from an illness, these foods can be easily ingested and blended into soups.

Fresh chicken, fish or seafood with lightly seasoned grains (rice-millet - cous cous - barley) mixed with seasonal vegetables

Minimal wild game, duck, rabbit, hare, venison with plenty of seasonal vegetables and natural fruit and berry sauces i.e. redcurrant, cranberry, orange and apple etc. plus a grain supplement, inc. vegetable and millet/rice/barley and side salads with celery, spring onions, watercress and fresh seasonal herbs, including any of the following:- rosemary, thyme, chervil, tarragon, chive, fennel, cumin, capers, nutmeg, clove, horseradish, wild thyme (serpolet), saffron and dandelion, parsley, basil etc. to aid digestion.

Occasional minimal quantities of organic meat, with plenty of seasonal vegetables and classic sauces i.e. Roast beef with horseradish - Roast Pork and apple sauce, Lamb with mint sauce or redcurrant jelly etc. These help the meat to be digested more easily. Always accompany with a grain food e.g. Roast beef with a wholemeal Yorkshire Pudding. Beef in a wholemeal pastry (en Croute). Roast pork with a sage/onion/garlic and wholemeal crumb stuffing etc. Always chew food well especially meat and protein.

One can replace animal protein by soya, tofu, pulses, such as lentils, chick peas, yellow and green dried peas etc. with recipes such as hummus, un-spicy dhals, cooked in seasonal vegetable soups and stews. Pulses and Soya are packed full of protein but must be GM free and organic.

Eat more green leafy vegetables, cabbage, greens, etc. in warmer weather and more root vegetables, carrots, turnips, swede etc. in colder times, always maintaining a reasonable balance of both all year round.

Only have organic salads in warm weather but ensure the ingredients to be as agricide free as possible due to the direct unchanged chemical content retained on the surface of the constituents of the salad. The same applies to all fresh fruit and vegetables.

Seasonal fruit to end a meal, will assist digestion by closing or yinnising the digestive system.

Super yin desserts of ice-cream, chocolate, citrus fruit, bananas etc. or with high sugar content i.e. meringues etc. can be a satisfying occasional treat for a special reason, being more readily processed by the body in warmer weather. In cold weather, enjoy baked fruit pies, inc. apple, blackcurrant, redcurrants, plums etc. made with wholemeal flour, untreated sugar/honey/raisins/currants etc..

Habitual Evening Meal: (Preferably eaten at least 3 hours before retiring).

Organic vegetable soups (avoid tomato) with rice and barley, more grain in cold weather, with occasional top up of seafood or white meat. Accompanied with wholemeal, rye or crisp breads.

Light pasta dishes and vegetables, vegetable risotto. Good quality 'light' Chinese or Indian Dishes with minimal spices and additives.

Organic seasonal fruit to help digestion.

Beverages:

Try to keep pure, filtered fluid to 1 –1.1/2 litres a day depending on activity including:- herb tea, good quality mineral water, organic seasonal fruit juices, clean uncomplicated alcohol, occasional organically produced tea and coffee preferably a.m.

Snacks:

Occasional comfort foods like whole grain snacks, biscuits etc. to accompany hot beverages, and alcohol, during the day or early evening, should be low in fat, sugar, salt, and additives.

Eat more before midday and less afterwards and try to avoid burdening the digestive system before retiring.

PART TWO

General Complaints

Allergies (including hay fever)

General Symptoms

Allergies are the collective term to describe symptoms of some people's reaction to allergens which come in several forms and are generally harmless. The most prevalent is Asthma which is dealt with in the next section. They can effect any age group. There are two main types of allergies, immediate or slow reacting ones. The instant reactive allergies cause substances from the immune system, such as histamine and leukotrienes, to be released into the body immediately. The delayed allergenic reactions like skin eruptions can take hours or several days to show. The immediate reactive allergies include hay fever, insect venom allergy, asthma, migraines, some food allergies caused by nuts and so forth. Some of these in certain persons can cause a most severe reaction of anaphylactic shock which derives from the Greek meaning 'ana'-excessive, 'phylaxis'- protection. Where the sufferer has difficulty in breathing and low blood pressure almost immediately after coming into contact with the allergen. This can be a drug, vaccine, insect bite or sting, chemicals, house dust, mites, pollution and some foodstuffs. One can have a varying degree of allergic reactions to chemicals found in carpets, furniture, paint, toxic waste etc.. The modern cocktail of chemicals and unnatural substances from all corners is on the increase, producing an ever-increasing level of allergies. They are multiplying on par with the growth of unnatural food aided and abetted by general pollution from food, air and water. The irony is that the consumer age has brought so many freedoms from old diseases and lifestyles only to impose a new set of curses for mankind.

Causes

Immediate reactive allergies are usually due to a weakened body defence mechanism. The body has two types of yang defensive chi, being an EMF field. It surrounds and circulates around the surface of the body protecting it from outer attack. This can clearly be seen as an aura in Kirlian photography. (*Please Refer* to ***Tai Chi Chuan & The Code of Life***). The inner one being the immune system. Both fed by the internal energy of the body. (*See* Part 3 on Chi Kung).

If the body is yinnised by habitat, diet or pathogens it will reduce both protective energy levels. The yang chi is yinnised by over consumption of yin foods, exposure to chemicals, radiation, electro-smogs and pollution. Also damp or wet environments are yin, contributing to the picture.

A yinnised person generally feels the cold more, tires more easily, as well as being prone to illness. Perhaps contributed to, by an inherited yin constitution. Both of which can be ameliorated. These types of allergies are exacerbated by an over consumption of yin substances to be found in industrialised foods which also weaken the immune system.

Triggers

Allergies can also be triggered by an excess of poor quality dairy food and animal protein. Modern dairy products contain many harmful additives such as antibiotics, hormones, chemicals and so forth which become concentrated into the foods, then passed on through the dairy produce into humans, where they slowly accumulate, until the system is overloaded and erupts. An additional cause is the abundance of cheap, tempting junk food permeated with chemical additives. The collective cocktail creating a climate for allergies which in truth is the body complaining; 'I cannot take any more of this rubbish'.

When the body reaches a yin peak, it fights back by reacting. It tries to defend itself against the alien substance by attacking the allergen.

The trigger could be animal fur, dust, mites, urban or countryside pollution, pollen, a bee sting, peanuts, chemicals etc.. The reaction severe or mild depends on how yin, the sufferer is. Histamine is the usual compound that is fed into the blood as the first line of defence. It is a yin substance derived from the amino acid, histidine. The DNA that makes up Histidine has the same binary code as Hexagram 49 from the I Ching. This hexagram 'Revolution' indicates a change taken from the idea of an animal moulting in response to the seasons. Oddly enough animal fur can be an allergen. (***Tai Chi Chuan & The Code of Life***).

An over secretion of histamine causes certain body tissue to dilate excessively especially smooth muscle of the lungs and in dire circumstances can cause anaphylactic shock. This is just a super yin reaction where the blood pressure is lowered with the lungs dilating. One emergency cure is to inject adrenaline which is very yang, to counter the allergic reaction, into the sufferer. Often bee keepers have adrenaline on hand as a protective measure.

The symptoms of the slower reactive allergies appear as eruptions on the skin, hair loss, rashes etc.. This is brought about excesses of yin or yang food, substances and lifestyle.

Internal Organs and Allergies

The excesses burden the organ of the kidney and its energy effects on the organism. This is caused by excess consumption of salty food and or poor quality dairy food, animal protein, acidic food and so forth. Thus the body's ability to cleanse itself by way of the kidneys is adversely affected. This is usually accompanied by a history of colds, flu, sore throats, damp hands and smelly feet. These are all signs of reduced kidney function. The kidneys eliminate a lot of toxins from the body and when these special hard working organs are overworked, the toxins are not displaced as easily. These waste products are re-circulated, being deposited on the skin as rashes, psoriasis and skin irritations also weakening the skin tissue. This can be exacerbated by exposure to chemicals and toxic substances. The inner toxins are then dumped on to the skin as a last resort, (*See* Skin Trouble Section). If one consumes too much yin or yang food and drink, these more gradual allergic reactions will occur. In Complementary Medicine (CM) the lung and large intestine are responsible for skin condition. It follows that if poor quality food is eaten regularly especially in childhood, the bowel will not function properly adversely effecting the skin as well as its sister organ of the lung. Cancer of the bowel and skin is exacerbated by industrialised foodstuffs.

The main contributor of slow allergic reactions is a continuous over indulgence of extremes of yin and yang food. Some general examples are, poor quality animal protein (yang) combined with alcohol (yin); salty foods whether natural or chemical (yang) balanced by spices (yin); savoury food like crisps (yang) as against 'sweet' drinks and sugar based confection (yin); cheese (yang) and tomato (yin); All these being unbalanced extremes, especially if the foods are highly industrialised, containing toxic additives.

Allergies as Warnings

Allergies are a warning of more serious illnesses to come, if the cause is not redressed.
The liver is another important organ that detoxifies. (*See* Detox Section). Liver function is greatly reduced by the pressure of too many toxins which stay in the bloodstream.

Sensitive skin should not be exposed to synthetic fibres or wool worn near the skin. Especially if cleaned in 'biological' or chemically harsh detergents. Always wash, the body, hair and clothes in safe mild 'eco-friendly' products. Man made fabrics can also irritate the skin, the safest material is cotton. Besides being an environmentally friendly fabric, it will relieve the skin from absorbing more unwanted chemicals through its pores. This harmful osmosis not only allows poisons to enter into the blood stream but prevents the skin from breathing, producing another vicious circle. The skin is the largest organ of the body.
Allergies are on the increase in line with pollutants from food, air and water. Many children are born with allergies due to this new pervasive factor inherited from the parents. Also a strong contributory factor is the lack of breast-feeding before weaning. It is recommended that a mother breast-feed her child for at least six months in order to protect it and build up its immune function and well being. Like any living entity the former years are the most important determining the quality of life in later years. Nevertheless the human condition has so many checks and balances, being able to change and adapt itself, it can easily redress most imbalances by adopting a balanced diet and lifestyle at most times in life. As allergies can be triggered by chemical substances, avoid exposure to the modern glues in furniture, foam backed carpets, paint, wall paper, aluminium saucepans, detergents and so forth.

Fillings

A hidden allergen is to be found in dental fillings made from amalgam. Grey dental amalgam is a by product of the ore of the metal mercury (*See* Teeth Section). Mercury is very yin and poisonous. In times gone by, many alchemical quacks tried to transmute mercury into gold. Only to be poisoned by the highly toxic vapour given off by the mercury, produced by their fruitless experiments. In the middle ages, compounds of liquid mercury were used as a cure for venereal disease, so called because it was considered as the affliction of passion or Venus. Mercury was considered a cure for this ailment, due to their planetary significance. The success of this dangerous preparation was precarious, for if too much mercury was taken, it could lead to madness and death.

Figure 1a: **The Kidney Meridian**

K1 The Bubbling Well Point - Yongquan - is so named, as it the point of entry of the yin chi of the earth into the foot and the beginning of the Kidney Meridian. The 'Kidney' is considered by Taoist Medicine to be the source of the 'Jing Chi' or life force of the organism. All mammals have this point.

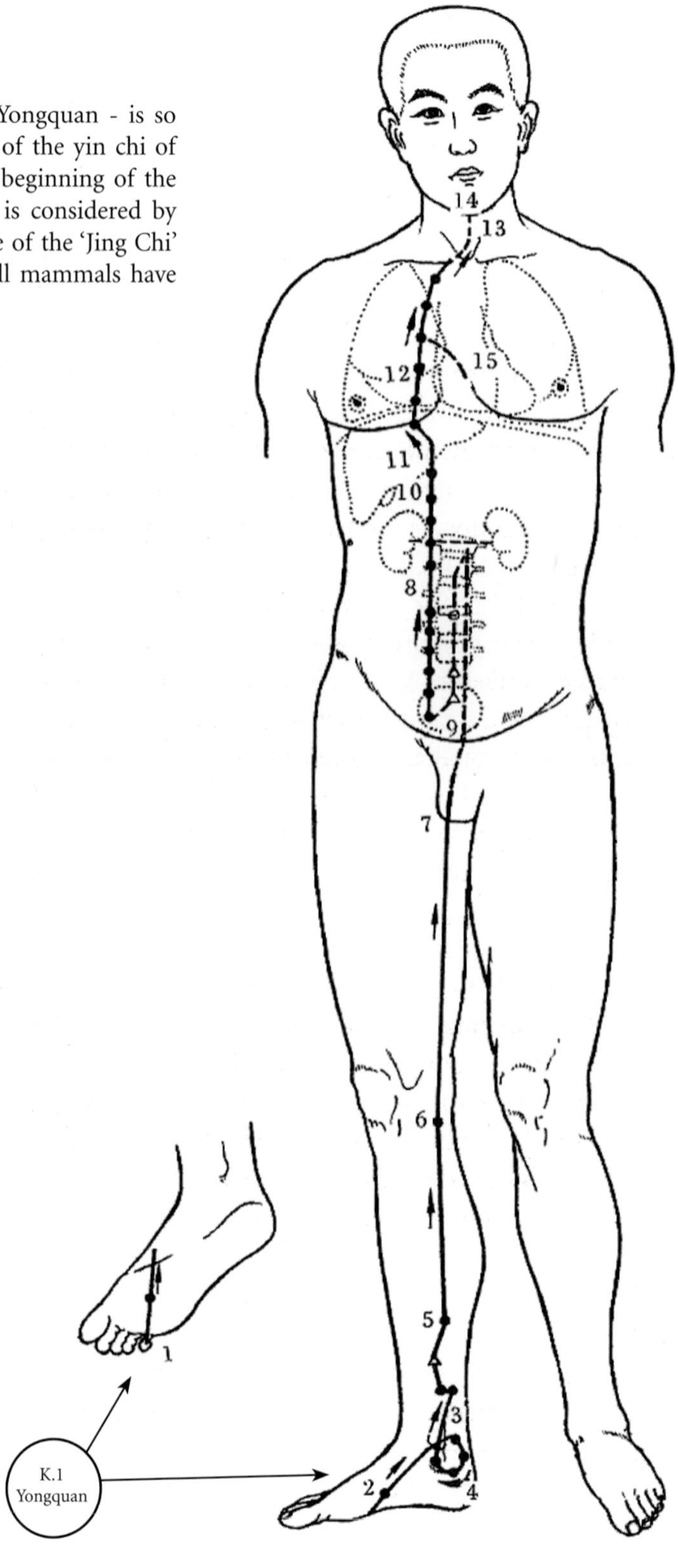

Emotional Response

Today the inner aspect of a human being is neglected in medicine. Most doctors only seeing the snap shot chemical symptoms of a person, overlooking the soul. Allergic reactions, slow or immediate can also be caused by emotional upsets, such as stress, bereavement, guilt, fear or anger. With symptoms erupting as skin rashes, hay fever, migraines or allergic reaction to foods.

For if a person suffers an unpleasant experience, synchronised at the same time as eating a certain food or a time of year and so forth, it can be experienced when the event, the food or season is encountered again, albeit negatively, causing an equivalent allergic reaction. This often happens in epilepsy that is not caused by tumours.

Even the Chinese Masters who founded Traditional Medicine, five thousand years ago, realised that there was an emotional response linked to each internal organ. For example if one suffers stress or fear, the internal energy of the kidney is unbalanced. It will slow down the kidney function reducing immune function, increasing toxin retention and effect will power. This form of diagnosis is empirical which I and many thousands of healers have used successfully over the centuries.

One will often find that the dietary cause is linked to the emotional cause. Both have to be treated equally. The inner disturbance can be uncovered by taking careful heed of dreams. Dreams are the objective voice of nature which will highlight the inconsistencies of our outer life. They achieve this by compensating the outer dilemmas with inner truths. Dr Jung proved this time and time again. One example is when he cured a long term asthmatic, in one session. He discovered the associated cause of the asthma in a dream. When the patient acknowledged this hidden trauma, it relieved the inner burden, thus taking the weight off the man's chest. However each soul being different, needing the unique individual approach which only the inner psyche can supply. At the centre of each person is the archetype of the Self, which has access to absolute knowledge.

An organic balanced yin yang diet will reconstitute the young very quickly because their internal energy is still expansive and yang i.e. engendering growth (*See* Part 1). If the allergies are allowed to continue or suppressed by drugs, the mother chi will be depleted prematurely. This will give rise to avoidable weakness in later life. If allergies persist in adults, after the age of thirty, they should be taken very seriously. The internal energy is waning with the body losing its ability to fight back. Therefore a strictly balanced yin yang diet of organic foods must be eaten until the allergy clears up, unaided by drugs, whenever possible.

Cure

Allergies are identified correctly by Western diagnostic techniques but in a superficial snap shot fashion. Western science and medicine sees the human condition as a chemical robot not realising the inter dependence of soul, mind and body. The specific allergens can be identified as chemicals, nuts, dust, pollen, nuts, strawberries, seafood etc.. However the real cause is overlooked which is that allergies are really a warning sign that the body is either too yin or yang.

This is usually due to an overload of toxins and if this situation is not addressed, will deplete the vital force of the body causing a steady decline over the ensuing years.

Although antihistamines and steroids are a quick fix for allergies. They are symptomatic, eventually reducing the immune function. This is the case for most synthetic substances, especially if taken over a long period. These toxins will over burden the kidneys and liver which naturally consider the drugs to be poisons, overloading the body's natural ability to cleanse itself.

The best way to rid oneself of allergies is to allow the organism to rest. It will permit the internal energy to balance. This is achieved safely by a centred natural diet free from all artificial additives, colouring and preservatives. This is laid out in the yin yang diet. To begin with cut out all habitual allergenic foods. After one has cleaned up the organism, one can test the healing process by experimenting with small amounts of the old taboo foods. Do not try foods outside of the suggested yin yang diet until really cured.

Hay fever is an overly yin condition provoked by excess yin. (*Refer* to Yin Yang Diet). Therefore one must try and reduce liquid intake to ½ - ¾ of clean, properly filtered fluid a day during the danger periods of superabundant atmospheric irritants like pollen. Excess liquid 'swills' around the body inflaming the mucous membranes of the nose, sinuses and the lungs which will react more aggressively when damp or yin. Spices, fruit, sugar confection will also yinnise and irritate these membranes. The reaction being the symptoms of the runny nose, sore eyes, coughing and sneezing etc.. Asthma is a yin complaint being an energy related cousin of hay fever. Therefore if one wants to completely heal the hay fever more quickly, one should follow the recommendations from the Asthma section.

Diet

Both immediate and slower allergy sufferers should detoxify the system by sticking to the yin yang diet. Immediate reactive allergic sufferers should reduce yin intake, whenever and wherever possible, taking special care to keep away from industrialised and junk foods which have additives, chemicals, preservatives. Hay fever is greatly assisted by moderating liquids, confection and spices. Keep pure liquid intake to sensible minimum of ½ - ¾ of a litre of clean fluids including the suggested herb teas below. Avoid all sweet food including honey, sugar and sugary products, diet drinks, dairy food, eggs and animal protein until better.

The slower reacting allergies of skin trouble should pay special attention to the quality and type of yang food including fish and animal protein. Preferably keeping to a vegetarian grain diet as suggested, supplemented by beans and pulses, with an emphasis on kidney beans.

Garlic besides strengthening the immune function aids the body to dispel toxins, helping to clear allergic reactions. Garlic is yin, therefore one clove a day is more than enough.

Herbs

Immediate reactive allergies being yin need yang to help counter the yin effect, good quality ginseng for males is helpful. Women should only take ginseng mixed with Royal Gelée.

Cleansing herbs can greatly help detoxify the body including the following:- echinacea, rosemary, thyme, chervil, celery, tarragon, chive, fennel, cumin, capers, nutmeg, clove, horseradish, wild thyme (serpolet), saffron and dandelion.

Herbs and plants that are helpful for the kidneys are fennel, parsley, chervil, tarragon, sage, burdock, bladderwort, dandelion and nettle.

Drinks which help detox the liver and gall bladder are infusions of rosemary, thyme, mint, meadowsweet, elderflower, decoction of artichoke and milk thistle as well camomile being also tonifying.

Exercise and Massage

Allergies are the body's way of fighting off toxins, needing the internal energy to be in harmony. (*Refer to* Part 3, Section 1 for reverse breathing). Do this exercise preferably early morning after rising and or early evening. This will increase lung power as well as stimulating and massaging the viscera. These Chi Kungs fortify the immune function by stimulating kidney energy. These deep breathing exercises will also boost the liver energy, assisting the detoxifying process. Also first thing after rising in the morning:-

1) Rub the ears gently forwards and backwards with the fingers, this will help 'wake up' and fortify the kidneys and their chi in the morning.

2) Gently tap the lower back over the kidney area with lightly clenched fists being very beneficial because it will stimulate 'kidney' essence.

3) K1 at the centre of the pad of the feet can be stimulated with a finger or by the heat of a lighted moxa herb bundle or even an incense stick.

4) Hay fever sufferers can help clear the sinuses, early morning before attacks set in by gently rubbing the hands together to produce friction chi. After which one places the middle joint of bent thumbs (digit 1) in the sinus cavities below the eyes next to the cheek bones. Then with the crook of the curved index fingers (digit 2) rub the upper sinuses in a semicircular fashion. The upper sinuses are situated over the eyebrows on the lower horizontal aspect of the forehead. The second stage of this massage is carried out by keeping the index fingers, firmly placed over the upper sinuses. After which one stimulates the lower sinuses, under the eye with the bent thumbs. This will attract chi and blood to flow around the sinuses, assisting the natural clearing of these areas. Rub gently as many times as you wish and do not be alarmed by the mucous discharge which will be relative to the amount stored up. This can cause sneezing which is the body's natural mechanism to expel negative yin energy including mucous. This will greatly help prevent the involuntary discharge of an attack, as the sinuses will be cleared of any excess mucous.

Always check with a medical practitioner if you are going to take herbal remedies whilst taking prescribed medicines.

Anaemia

Diagnosis

A general guide to check for anaemia is lack of vitality, breathlessness, loss of sexual libido accompanied by whitish fingernails, white colour on inside of lower eyelids, grey or whitish lips and pale cheeks. A blood test can confirm this.

Nutritional Anaemia

Cause

Nutritional anaemia, is a deficiency of iron, cobalt, copper, various proteins and vitamins such as B-12. A lack of haemoglobin reduces oxygen absorption producing the anaemic symptoms. Although most health care specialists prescribe iron supplements there is a natural long term solution.

However the body can synthesise iron naturally from a balanced yin yang diet. A lack of chlorophyll in the diet due to a reduced intake of green leafy vegetables, and an over consumption of yin type foods accompanied by yin environments will cause anaemia. Iron is at the core of haemoglobin being the basis of all animal life which also eat plant material, yet having healthy iron levels. For example large animals such as cows, bulls and giraffes are naturally healthy on a plant diet. So can humans be. The basis of plant life is magnesium, a lack of which in the diet causes the iron deficiency, however the body can also synthesise iron from magnesium. There a vast populations in Asia who for centuries have been vegetarian without having anaemia, however their diet relates to their climate and must be adjusted for a change in environment. (*Refer to* Yin Yang principles in Part 1).

Long Term Cure

It is more natural and a longer term solution to eat an organic diet comprising of c. 65% grains, soya and bean protein balanced by a 35% intake of fresh green, leafy vegetables which are in season, such as kale, seaweed, daikon (white radish) leaves, watercress, cabbage, sprouts, etc.. Grain foods help assimilate the iron and or magnesium from leafy greens which also contain the anti-oxidant Vitamin C. Chlorophyll is naturally transmuted into iron by all mammals including humans. An elephant does not eat meat or need iron supplements in the wild yet produces iron naturally from the plant based magnesium found in its natural habitats. Magnesium is the basis of chlorophyll. Thus haemoglobin and chlorophyll are synergistic.

Herbs

Herbs that help are Echinacea, although only to be taken for a short time, increases red blood cells- (pregnant mothers should limit Echinacea intake to a ¼ dosage for a week only), mugwort/wormwood dandelion, gentian, hops, nettles and all of which can be taken as teas.

Organic miso and tamari being fermented vegetable foods contain B-12 as well as seaweeds, all of which help the magnesium/iron synthesis.

Pernicious Anaemia

Michio Kushi considers that pernicious anaemia is caused by a lack of B-12, thus a yin yang diet with a focus on the above accompanied by an emphasis of organic miso vegetable soup taken every morning will relieve this.

Sickle Cell Anaemia

Kushi also considers sickle cell anaemia which is prevalent amongst Afro-Caribbeans and Black Americans to be caused by an overly yin diet. This exacerbates the predisposition of the sickle cell which evolved to counter malaria in Africa. A balanced yin yang diet will counter the effect of this genetic mechanism from becoming aggressive. The sickle cell is yin whereas the red blood cell is yang, thus a junk food diet littered with yin chemicals will create a yin condition allowing this genetic defence to go awry causing the symptoms of this disease to manifest.

Taboos

Avoid spinach because it contains oxalic acid which leaches as well as inhibits iron from the body as do tomatoes, aubergines, egg plant, rhubarb and potatoes. Also stay away from yin foods such as sugar, soft drinks, sodas, alcohol, drugs, spices, junk food etc.. (*See* Yin Yang Diet).

Quick Fix Iron Foods

There are dietary quick fixes of foods that are rich in iron and can be found in red meat, pig's liver, egg yolks, dried peaches, apricots, nuts, oysters, raw clams, lentils, molasses, oatmeal, prunes and beans. Traditional cooking in ironware is also a simple way of putting iron into the diet.

If you wish to buy iron as a supplement, the RDA is 10-18 mgs per day, pregnant and lactating woman need 30-60 mgs per day. It is best to buy a natural source in liquid form of hydrolised-protein chelate, an organic iron which has been processed for quick assimilation.

Exercise

Plenty of fresh clean air coupled with rhythmic aerobic stimulating movement will help. During pregnancy walking and non strenuous cycling are good, plus - Chi Kung 1a-b), 2), 3), 5), 6), 7) & 8) - (Pregnant women should only do 1a-b), 2)). Tai Chi is also excellent as oxygen absorption is maximised without physical stress during these gentle stimulating movements as well. Tai Chi and Chi Kung will stimulate the bone marrow which is an area of red blood cell production, also the small intestine where red blood cells are made in conjunction with other parts of the organism can be stimulated by massage and reverse breathing.

Conclusion

Anaemia is a symptom of chaotic or erratic eating which in turn is an effect of neglect of the mind and body. This can be caused by rejection, depression amongst other disturbances of the spirit which needs focus as well. (*Refer* to the section on Stress). Therefore diet plus a release of inner tension is required to allow a wholesome cure.

Always check with a medical practitioner if you are going to take herbal remedies whilst taking prescribed medicines.

Asthma

General Symptoms and Causes

Asthma is generally caused by an overly 'yin' condition or expansive state (*See* Yin Yang Diet). The lungs are a yin organ performing effectively when the tissues are 'compact' or 'yang'. Therefore a diet which is too yin will cause the lungs to become over dilated causing the air passages of the lung to swell and restrict breathing. The tightness of the chest and the coughing associated with asthma is caused by spasm in the bronchial tubes and or by secretion of excessive amounts of mucous trapped in the airways. These are the result of excesses of yin energy from food, unnecessary use of anti-biotics by a gestating mother or in early childhood, exacerbated by the dust, pollen, house mites etc. and a polluted environment.

Yin substances encourage 'dampness' in the body as opposed to yang which engenders dryness. Excess yin has a tendency to over dilate body tissue thus expanding and constricting the linings of the lungs. Whereas a correct counter balance of yang energy will allow the lungs to operate properly by keeping the bronchi compact giving rise to open airways. Therefore a balance of yin and yang energies from diet, environment and lifestyle will naturally harmonise or heal the asthma and redress the effects of the excess yin. A natural healing process will also depend on the length and damage of the asthma, but as lungs are living tissue most cases of asthma, if not cured will be radically improved.

Asthma and The Internal Organs

Asthma sufferers have raised shoulders at acupoint (Lu.5) where the two lung channels of the acupuncture meridians, commence. The raised shoulders are caused by the disturbed energy or chi of the lung and acupoint (Lu.5) not only in the lung itself but also the associated meridians and brother organ in this case being the large intestine. The quality of the large intestine depends on the quality of the diet. An inactive bowel is often caused by excess yin food, especially industrialised foodstuffs. For example if food contains pesticide residues which are nerve inhibitors designed to kill insects, this effect also kills the healthy bacteria and flora of the intestine. This results in serious IBS problems and cancer as well, causing imbalance in the lung. The lung and large intestine are governed by the metaphoric element of 'metal' in Complementary Medicine. Just as metal can expand and contract so do the lungs and the intestines. These organs also control the energy of the skin and body hair as originally cited in the wisdom of an ancient Chinese medical canon. Asthma sufferers often have eczema and skin rashes echoing the 5000 year old Huang Ti Ni Ching.

Asthma is a general yin condition which can be more troublesome, if it is accompanied by an inherited yin constitution, giving rise to all the childhood chesty complaints aggravated by an overly yin diet or allergens. Any or all of the following can provoke asthma such as dust, animal fur, pollen, emotional disturbance, fatigue, cold air, smoke, damp or wet climates, anti-biotics, lack of or excess exercise, usual town pollution, country pollution from farm agro-chemicals as well as detergents on clothes. Most of these are yin catalysts.

Often asthmatic children on reaching puberty will rid themselves of this yin complaint as puberty is the start of the yang maturation of a human being, as well as the debacle of the

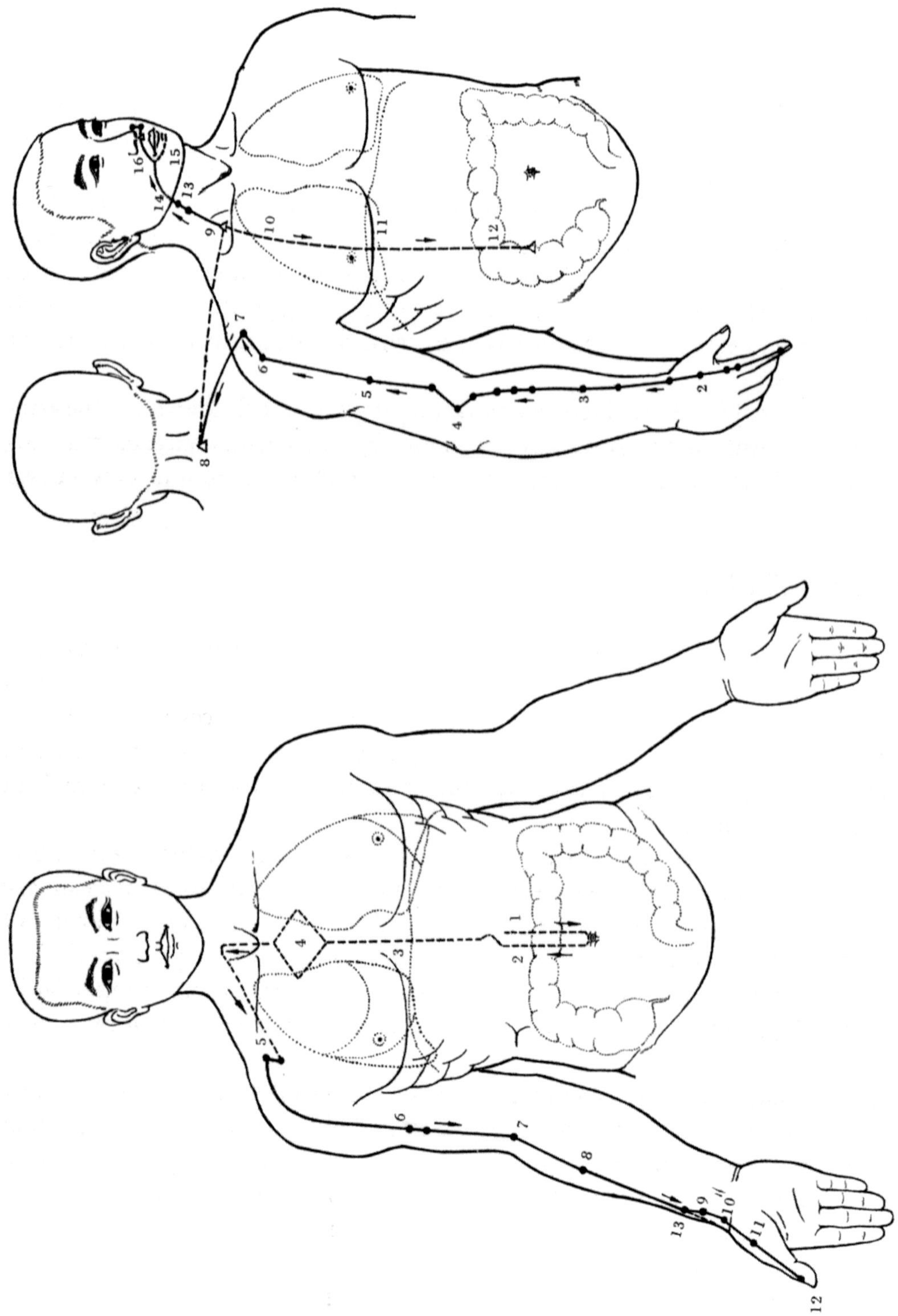

Figure 2: Course of the Lung Meridian; Course of the Large Intestine Meridian

yang outward expansion and separation of offspring from parental control.

Another reason for asthma is the relative body weight which has a bearing on respiration. Unnecessary bulk burdens the cardiovascular system which can create or intensify breathing difficulties.

Cure

Asthma is treated by conventional medicine with bronchodilators and nebulisers which widen the air passages by chemically 'relaxing' the bronchial smooth muscle. Although this gives temporary relief, it will actually worsen the yin asthma, as the drugs are also very yin. Also there are the unpleasant side effects caused by the drugs which have to be filtered out by the liver and kidneys. If these strong drugs are taken over a long period they will inhibit and damage vital organs, with residual symptoms of weight gain, thinning of the bones, high blood pressure, stomach ulcers, water retention and even stunting growth in children. A vicious circle is engaged because the sufferer has to increase the drug dose to counteract the inevitable side effects.

Natural methods applying the principles of yin and yang can cure the lungs and the asthma quite quickly. Firstly the lungs are 'yangised' naturally by centring the diet, thus removing excess yin from the body as well as avoiding damp and polluted environments whenever possible.

Yin and Yang and The Lungs

The lung is an 'air' sponge, being a very fine sensitive yin organ designed to discharge CO_2 which is the yang by-product of the body and absorb O_2 which is the yin elixir of life from plants and trees. Therefore besides a balanced diet one must reduce excess yin intake, especially liquids. An asthmatic should reduce uncomplicated fluids to ½ - ¾ a litre a day. Also ensuring a daily regime of clean fresh air, from dry natural environments, preferably in countryside, parks, seaside etc..

A natural way to ease an asthma attack is firstly to stay as calm as possible in a pollution free zone away from dust, animals, pollen etc.. Then before or during an attack one can take a spoonful of sesame salt, sometimes called 'Gomasio'. This is 1 part sea salt to 10 parts of washed and dried, 'roasted' organic sesame seeds, ground together, naturally if possible. The sesame salt being yang will help to close the bronchioles and so ease the air passages. Sucking a piece of good quality ginseng root or a tablet will also ease an attack for the same yang reason.

These yang substances will help contract the alveoli, the terminal air sacs of the lungs, thus freeing the airways to their natural biological condition. A child is born with about 20,000,000 alveoli and an adult has about 300,000,000 of these microscopic blind-ended sacs where the exchange of CO_2 and O_2 take place. When this microscopic sensitive tissue is yinnised, it swells up, preventing the air from passing into the system. When it is yangised, it contracts, freeing these vital air passages, allowing O_2 to pass freely into the body.

A daily regimen of rinsing and brushing the mouth and teeth with very fine sea salt will yangise the saliva helping to yangise the system. It will also act as an excellent gum fortifier as well as reducing oral bacteria in the mouth.

One must be careful not to overdo salt consumption as it can reduce kidney function, raising blood pressure.

Besides reducing liquid intake one must eat 'dry' foods, avoiding boiled and or wet soggy foods, trying to eat grains and vegetables which have been baked, grilled or fried. In Complementary Medicine, the Large Intestine is the brother organ of the lung and if it is in poor condition it will drain away vital energy from the lung chi. To keep the large intestine in good shape always eat plenty of roughage in the form of organic whole grains, such as brown rice, wholemeal bread, sweet corn etc.. Season with sesame salt (gomasio). (*Refer to* Yin Yang Diet). Keep away from fruit and salads as although roughage, they are too yin for asthmatics.

Keep to a diet of 60% yang foods comprising of 'dry' cooked whole cereal grains (*See* Yin Yang Diet); 20% pulses; 15 % yang vegetables, including plenty of yang 'dry' cooked vegetables especially cauliflower, broccoli, leafy greens and carrots, turnips, swede, green beans, peas, onions etc.. ***Avoid tomatoes, spinach, aubergine and potatoes***; 5% liquid intake in the form of filtered water and or herb teas, like peppermint, refrain from regular coffee, tea, cold or iced drinks. The taboo foods to avoid are dairy products (cheese, milk, butter and eggs), fruit, salads, spices, ice cream, confection, junk food and any food that has additives, preservatives, colouring and so forth.

Herbs and Plants that are helpful for the lungs are:- thyme, rosemary, fennel, parsley, garlic, chervil, liquorice, mint and celery. Lobelia can also be used as a vasodilator.

Massage

The back and chest can be massaged with essential oils of eucalyptus, lavender and thyme; especially at each of the hollows cited below the extremities of the collar (clavicle) and arm (humerus) bones, at lung meridian Pts. (Lu.5 & 6) (*fig.2*). Also along the vertical hollow of the sternum at the centre of the breast bone Pts. (CV.16/17/18). For an easy and constant therapeutic stimulus of the lung chi and its meridian one can press at (Lu.12) of both thumbs (digit1) with the tips of the index fingers (digit2), on the radial side of the thumb (digit1), next to the lowest corner of the nail. These oils can be vaporised in burners to help sufferers and ease attacks at night and so forth. These acupoints not only can ease an attack but are a constant aid, increasing lung energy.

Exercise and Breathing

Always try and breath through the nose during the day and whilst sleeping. When feeling able, learn to hold one's breath from time to time, extending the period until reaching about 30 seconds. This can be done whilst walking, sitting or doing Chi Kung. These simple tips will ease the bronchi and help prevent seizures but not cure the asthma. This principle has been exploited by a Russian called Konstantin Buteyko who realised that the lungs would 'close' down if they held too much oxygen. He noticed that when one retains carbon dioxide by holding the breath, it allowed the lungs to relax. This method can temporarily free the air passages thus alleviating an attack. His method has achieved success in Russia, Australia and New Zealand. However he does not explain how this method works or the causes of the asthma.

The cause of asthma and his method can be explained easily by applying the energy concepts of yin and yang.

Oxygen is yin and if retained in excess in the lung, accompanied by poor shallow breathing will over yinnise an already 'yinnised' yin organ. It makes the air passages expand giving rise to an attack. Whereas carbon dioxide is yang, making the lungs contract, thereby opening the bronchi and relieving the spasm. Buteyko with his extensive research, had inadvertently come across and exploited the natural law of yin yang.

His system at the outset can be a useful tool to produce a 'self-help' mind set and all too welcome respite. However it will not root out the underlying cause, but produce a window of opportunity to aid the healing process. The cure has to address diet, environment and stress.

When an asthma attack is felt coming on, try and remove oneself from any allergens and sit or stay still, slightly hollowing the chest and do the reverse breathing in Part 3. One must learn to keep the thoughts as calm as possible. Also making affirmative statements to oneself like: 'I am in control, neither do I want nor will I have an attack'. Above all stay tranquil and relaxed as possible.

Hence the asthmatic posture of the raised shoulders is akin to the fright posture, albeit for different reasons, for when the internal energy is upset it produces an upward, destabilising result.

Therefore when the sufferer realises he or she has gained more self-control, the fear of an attack will dissolve, just as any problem which once faced, loses its sinister power. If this procedure is repeated the mind body association will go from strength to strength, allied with the diet and the other suggestions can cure the asthma completely.

Plenty of good quality 'fresh' air in dry natural environments is a tonic plus learning to breath with the diaphragm. Make it a regular precautionary regimen to fortify the respiratory system by doing 'reverse breathing'. It is an excellent way to increase oxygen intake, reinforcing the lungs as well as massaging the vital organs. Deep breathing should be carried out early morning, in clean pollution free environments preferably in natural surrounding near trees or the sea etc.. (*See* Part 3, Chi Kung Section 1.)

Another strengthening Chi Kung for the Lung and Large Intestine, is to firstly fire up the chi by reverse breathing with joined hands (right over left for the female, vice versa for the male). The joined palms covering the Tan Tien, (CV.6) *(fig.14)* situated about two inches below the navel.

Then remove one hand only and place it on the Mingmen Gate (GV.4) *(fig.14)* sited at the space between the kidneys between the 2nd and 3rd lumbar vertebrae. Return the hand to the Tan Tien for 'charging', then repeat with the other hand and so forth. Repeat in blocks of 4 breaths

Also one can rub the hands to produce friction chi then place a flat palm over the centre of the chest area, then with the palm of the other hand rub in a circular fashion around the abdomen over the position of the large intestine. Do this in both a clockwise and anticlockwise manner symmetrically, alternating the hands, preferably early morning or whenever convenient. The above exercises can be accompanied by 2) from Part 3.

Always check with a medical practitioner if you are going to take herbal remedies whilst taking prescribed medicines.

Back and Neck Pain

General Symptoms and Causes

Backache and neck ache are pain along the spine or muscles of the back, caused by muscle strain or other muscular disorders, pressure on the root of a nerve, or a ruptured vertebral disk. The superficial damage to these parts of the anatomy is due to blockages or disturbances of energy that run up and down the back. There are two main sources of internal energy, chi, that support this area of the muscular and skeletal frame. Firstly is the flow of internal energy which courses through the bladder meridian supplied and augmented by chi of the Governing vessel, the Dumo (*fig.14*). The bladder meridian runs up either side of the Dumo. The bladder meridian is a bifurcated channel, about five centimetres apart, with the Governing vessel sitting in the middle along the spine. These channels feed energy to the muscles and spine on their journey up and down the back. The energy of the Dumo runs up and down, whereas the chi of the bladder meridian runs down.

Wherever chi is restricted, blocked or disturbed, the corresponding area of influence around the meridian, is weakened, in this case the spine and back. The weakness in this region is usually brought to an acute condition by sport, bad posture, an accident and so forth. The bladder meridian is disturbed for a variety of reasons quite often when its mother organ is over burdened by too much liquid and acidic food and drink and yin substances. (*Refer to* Yin Yang Diet).

There is a secondary chi supply for the muscles (tendons) and bones which is conditioned indirectly by the liver and kidney chi respectively. If the liver is overloaded (*Refer to* Detox Section) the chi that feeds the muscles is interfered with. Also if the kidney chi is disturbed (*See* Yin Yang Diet and Chi Kung Sections) the strength of the bones and joints is affected. Poor diet, anger, fear or shock and stress will also disturb chi flow in these organs, thereby effecting the corresponding muscles and skeletal structure.

Posture

Another contributory factor, which puts tension and causes pain in the back, is posture related. This is due to internal energy flow differentials from inherited as well as traumatic factors like a blow or a fall etc..

If we take a Complementary Medicine view of the body that the feet are the weight bearing stand of the body acting like the foundations of a building. It is easy to compare the structural problems of both by working our way up from the base. So if the root energy is disturbed, by having one foot or usually leg longer than the other, it will upwardly effect the whole skeletal structure including the back and spine. This vital area being a long section of bone with many supporting muscles which when disturbed by poor posture or erratic chi flow etc. will put this upright part of our survival in jeopardy. One should always maintain a good stance that adheres and augments the natural flow of chi. (*Refer to* Central Equilibrium in Part 3, for the chi aligned posture). The single weighted or 'one legged' Chi Kung from this section will correct postural defects with continued practice.

Stress:

The energy of the back can also be interfered with by stress. In Complementary Medicine the back represents the past and often damage to the area that is behind one, is induced by a bad experience also from the past. The back is also the part of the anatomy that keeps one upright. So when the back buckles, it can be a burden from the past that is too much to bear.

I had an Asian patient, a gentle young man who could never straighten his neck. He was constantly dipping his head like a chicken. It was as if he was split in two, one side saying to him 'stand up', whilst the other pressed down on his neck. I discovered the trouble to be that his father, the family patriarch, died during an inter family dispute, when he was quite young. As the eldest son he had to become the head of the family and try to resolve these burdensome, family issues. The neck became an outer manifestation of the inner conflict. Hence the desire to straighten countered by the psychological pressure of being unable to cope with this load.

Often I have patients who have a pain in the neck because they have a relationship that is a pain in the neck. The mind can interfere with the flow of energy in a very direct and obvious way.

Cure

Centring the organism is important with any complaint to permit healing to take place. The energy that feeds the meridians of the back will be harmonised by a balanced diet, allowing any damage to heal properly, for the long term. The chi, that flows through meridians of the back, is disturbed by excess yin intake. The excess yin is usually incorrectly counter balanced by an indulgence of poor quality yang foods. These extremes stress the internal energy causing a vicious circle. No matter how much remedial exercise or treatment is done to strengthen and align the back, it will not be cured until the underlying weakness in the energy system is breached. When the energy is clear, the spine and back can be realigned, healing the symptoms of the painful pulled muscles, slipped discs, torticollis and so forth.

The remedies for back and neck complaints are greatly assisted by adopting the Central Equilibrium posture from Part 3, as well as Chi Kung and massage. These external factors must be combined with removing the excess yin and toxins from the body by toning up the kidney and the bladder chi, which is the root energy cause.

Therefore try to keep pure fluid intake to ½-¾ litre a day, albeit relative to fluid loss, but to free these channels it is best to keep away from heavy exercise until the back or neck are better. Never expose the back or neck to damp or cold, always keep them covered and warm. Saunas and steam baths will help dry out the excess liquid from the body as well as opening the chi channels of the spine and dispelling toxins from the body and muscles. When sleeping try and stay lying on one's back as much as possible with a firm mattress. Keep the spine supported and straight with minimal pillow support. At work whether passive or active, ensure that the spine is kept upright even when lifting or working at a desk. All these factors will assist the chi to run freely again through the effected channels and permit healing to take place and restore the back and neck to its natural state.

When balancing diet with the yin yang principles one must pay special attention to reducing liquid intake to ½ - ¾ a litre a day, steering clear from dairy food, spices, heavy animal

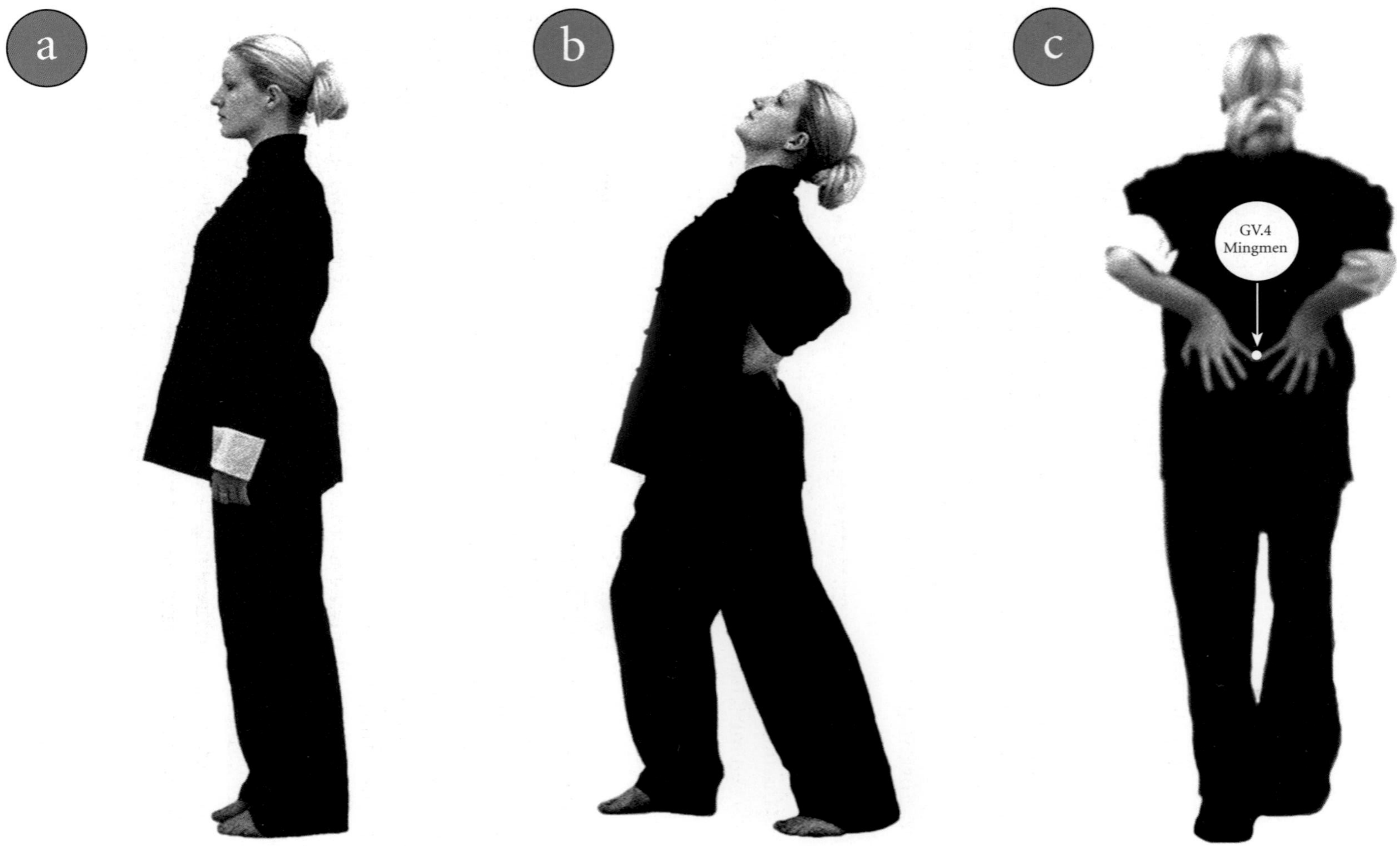

Figure 3: **The Bridge** - The Bridge exercise works on various levels. Besides easing and rectifying back pain, it will act to strengthen the back by ensuring that the chi is free to flow in the salient meridians, thus fortifying the muscles in that area, preventing any potential back trouble as well as a cure. Remember diet plays an important part in energy balancing. Firstly breath in as you step forward with hands as in C) and gently arch your back supported by your hands, as far as you can go comfortably, as in B). Then exhale as you relax and return to the neutral position of A). Repeat x4 off each leg.

protein, red meat and tropical fruit especially bananas, mangoes, citrus fruits and their like if you live in a temperate climate.

Diet

Keep to a diet of **60%** yang foods comprising of 'dry' cooked whole cereal grains, (*See* Yin Yang Diet), **20%** pulses, **10%** yang vegetables, **5%** indigenous fruit in season (not acidic), **5%** pure liquid intake (½-¾ a litre a day) in the form of uncomplicated fluids including, filtered water, herb teas like burdock and dandelion, nettle, keeping away from regular coffee or tea. Reduce all alcohol especially wine and spirits. Try to avoid all dairy foods (cheese, milk, butter and eggs), spices, confection, junk food and food that have additives, preservatives, colouring and so forth.

Grain foods such as brown rice and buckwheat are good for the digestion and circulation, plus all the whole grain foods, to add variety, are acceptable. Try and keep yeasted whole wheat breads to a minimum, it is preferable to have the unleavened breads until the system ameliorates.

The pulses and beans that are good for kidneys are the kidney beans, aduki beans and mung beans.

Vegetables like carrots, celery, turnips, swede, cauliflower, beans, broccoli, leeks, onions and greens etc.. ***Try avoiding tomatoes, spinach, aubergine and potatoes.***

Herbs and Plants that are helpful for the kidneys are fennel, parsley, chervil, tarragon, sage, burdock, bladderwort, dandelion, nettle, Devil's Claw, ginseng and valerian.

Massage

Also to alleviate lower back trouble, one can energise and free the area by gently rubbing up and down either side of the spine as far as one can reach, producing 'friction' chi. Chi flows more readily in warm conditions. In summer, energy circulates more readily through the channels nearer to the surface of the body. Whereas in winter the chi is naturally slower and deeper. If the pain is severe, the area can be massaged by a third party, with an active rubbing balm or enlivening essential oils of rosemary, pine, thyme, lavender, as well as Tiger Balm along the course of the bladder meridian and Governing Vessel. This should be carried out in an upward motion from the base of the spine up to the neck. Also massage the sore area anticlockwise to reduce swelling, with the idea of activating the chi back to the area.

The aforementioned herbs as well as sea salt and seaweed, can be used in hip baths morning and night to assist circulation of blood and energy.

To invigorate the Kidney and Triple Heater channels, rub, in a stroking motion with both hands down the outside (yang) of the legs and then back up towards the body on the inside (yin) of the legs. Then with one hand rub, in a stroking motion outward away from the body along the outside of the arm (yang) and back up towards the body on the inside of the arm.

Lightly tapping the lower back with clenched fists early morning after rising will tone kidney and bladder chi and function as well as easing back pain. A painful neck can be relieved by gentle friction, with finger massage, using the same oils mentioned above, in vertical and horizontal strokes up and around the neck.

To assist the healing and help straighten the spine go to a qualified chiropractic and ask him or her to align the vertebrae if necessary which will speed up the process.

Exercise and Breathing

If the muscles of the back have gone into spasm one has to rest and wait for the muscles to ease before doing any exercise. The following exercise, called the bridge, can be done even if there is still local pain as the hands act like the supports of a bridge.

Stand with one leg in front of the other and place both palms on the lower back, over the kidney area, elbows tucked in as much as possible. Then whilst breathing in, one arcs the supported spine by bending backwards, looking as far back as possible. On the out breath one returns to an upright position, repeat on the other leg. Carry out in blocks of four (*fig.3*).

A general exercise to tone up the muscles of the lower back if there is no acute pain, is to lie on one's back, palms flat on the floor with arms pointing straight down in line with the torso, supporting the body. Raise the legs one inch off the floor with a slow in breath, hold for a split second, then gently exhale whilst lowering the legs. As the back muscles become stronger one can raise the legs higher and more slowly on the in breath, until one reaches a ninety-degree angle, then lowering the limbs during exhalation. The next stage is to inhale with the legs raised as above then with the legs at a ninety degree angle. Then open like a pair of scissors sideways, on the out breath, after which one takes an in breath whilst drawing the legs back to their upright position. Finally exhaling as the legs are lowered to the ground.

Even when the back is painful one can do a variety of Chi Kungs from Part 3 whilst lying down flat on one's back to assist chi circulation and aid recovery: being 1), 2), 3), 7) & 8).

Once the back is becoming stronger one can do appropriate amounts of one legged Chi Kung which permits the spine to be aligned without the need for the back to compensate for one leg being longer than the other. Different leg length and weak ankles can be a major reason for bringing about back trouble. If one avoids 'double weighted stances' it will greatly improve the overall posture relieving unnecessary pressure from the spine and neck. Take special attention to adhere at all times to the Central Equilibrium posture from Part 3, and perform a variety of the following:-

1), 2), 3), 4), 6), 7), 8) & 9). These will not only strengthen the back and neck but also stimulate the whole organism.

The neck has to support the head which weighs about ten to twelve pounds in an average adult. Thus making an upright posture and correct neck alignment a necessity. Ensure one holds the head directly above the spine without leaning in any way, whilst sitting, standing at work or play. Again neck weakness is related to the flow of chi in several meridians which support the muscles that hold up the head. If the chi around the neck is healthy there is less chance of damage or hurt, but when these muscles have been pulled, still try and keep the head as upright as possible. If need be wearing a brace to ensure alignment whilst healing is taking place. A burden on the liver and gallbladder organs and their chi can weaken the neck area as their meridians run along the neck and the side of the head. A disruption in these meridians also cause migraines and headaches for the same reason.

When on the road to recovery there are four general exercises to strengthen the neck, the cervical vertebrae and its muscles. Maintaining the Central Equilibrium posture and carry out in blocks of four:

a) Roll the head in a large circle around on an in breath and back around the other way on the out breath.

b) Breath in and point the head down chin on chest. Whilst exhaling, gently take the head back as far as it will go.

c) Breath in whilst turning and keeping the head to the left in a horizontal plane and exhale on returning the head to face forward, repeat to the right.

d) Breath in and bend the head to the left, directing the left ear towards the left shoulder, exhale on straightening the head, repeat the other side.

A good time to carry out energy exercises is early morning or less effectively, when the chi is charging the kidney and bladder meridians, between 3.00p.m. to 5.00p.m. and 5.00p.m to 7.00p.m. respectively. (GMT/UK or local solar time).

The Bridge exercise works on various levels. Besides easing and rectifying back pain, it will act to strengthen the back by ensuring that the chi is free to flow in the salient meridians, thus fortifying the muscles in that area, preventing any potential back trouble as well as a cure. Remember diet plays an important part in energy balancing.

Always check with a medical practitioner if you are going to take herbal remedies whilst taking prescribed medicines.

Cellulite

General Symptoms and Causes

There are many misconceptions about cellulite, however it is basically fatty deposits which the body naturally tends to retain in specific areas for later use, especially in women. It is an evolutionary left over, acting as an organic storage failsafe. This natural mechanism to conserve is more crucial in women for building up vital reserves for childbearing and breastfeeding. One of the main places it shows in the female is around the waist, buttocks, thighs and legs. The pithy effect of cellulite is more predominant in women, because female skin tissue is thinner and the fibres are more taught than with men, making the fatty deposits dimple like an orange peel. Whereas fatty tissue in men is more evenly distributed due to a looser and thicker skin tissue. Cellulite is intensified by an inactive lifestyle, poor circulation and an unbalanced diet.

Personal Blight of Cellulite

Just like every person every complaint is fairly unique. Therefore some women are more prone than others to show these fatty deposits in certain regions of the body. Basically cellulite is caused by the pressure on the liver which is burdened by excess yin foodstuffs. The main antagonists being alcohol, chocolate, sweets, excess fats and oils, normal commercial margarine and 'butter replacement' spreads, high sugar content foods and soft drinks, diet drinks (the sugar free additives are as bad if not worse as the sugar they replace because they contain many chemical additives which also reduce liver function), industrialised foods with chemical additives. Also included in the list are the inept foodstuffs like spices, spinach, tomatoes, potatoes, tropical fruit and vegetables, in other words all extreme yin varieties of foodstuffs. This pressure on the body can be exacerbated by the combined overeating of fatty foods, dairy foods and animal fat found in lamb, bacon, pork, suet, butter, cream, ice-cream, including junk food.

Overworked Liver

The complicated chemical functions of the liver are unique and it is the only organ function that modern medicine cannot synthesise mechanically. However it is the organ that can regenerate itself. Amongst its many functions is its ability to metabolise (break down) proteins, carbohydrates, and fats; stores glycogen, vitamins, and other substances as well as synthesising blood-clotting factors. It also removes wastes and toxic matter from the blood; regulates blood volume; and destroys old red blood cells. The liver is very essential to life, weighing in at 3-4 lbs. the same as the brain. The hard working liver operates in tandem with the kidneys and bladder to balance and clean the blood of waste products. Thus the surplus fatty acids which are not eliminated will be deposited as fat around the body.

The liver cells also synthesise a number of enzymes. As blood flows through the liver, both from the portal vein and from the hepatic artery, the cells and enzymes filter out and modify many substances and particles. Nutrients entering the liver from the intestine are changed into forms usable by the body cells or are stored for future use. Fats are converted into fatty acids and then into carbohydrates or ketone bodies and transported by the blood to the tissues, where they are further metabolised. Sugars are converted into glycogen, which remains stored in the liver until it is needed for energy production, then it is reconverted into glucose and released into the bloodstream. The liver manufactures blood serum proteins, including albumin and several clotting factors, and supplies them to the blood. In its role as a blood purifier, the liver metabolises nitrogenous waste products, urea, from body processes and detoxifies poisonous substances, preparing them for elimination in the urine or faeces. So as cellulite is linked to poor liver function it is also a warning of dire possibilities ahead if not redressed.

The Brother Gall Bladder

Its brother organ in Complementary Medicine, the gall bladder produces bile, also called 'gall', a greenish yellow secretion that is produced in the liver and passed to the gallbladder for concentration, storage, or transport into the first region of the small intestine, the duodenum. Its function is to aid in the digestion of fats in the duodenum. Bile is composed of bile acids and salts, cholesterol, pigments, water, and electrolyte chemicals that keep the total solution slightly acidic (with a pH of about 5 to 6).

The yang gallbladder and its sister yin organ of the liver help control weight because they control the digestion or retention of fatty substances in the body. So if these organs are under stress, weight can increase. This in turn over burdens the kidney function therefore water retention is increased giving rise to such symptoms as possibly swollen feet, ankles, legs, hands, wrists and 'puffy' face etc..

Quick and Simple Liver/Gall Bladder Test

The eyes are controlled by liver and gall bladder chi. A 'quick' liver test is to gauge how sensitive the eyes are to bright or strong light at night, or direct sunlight. This is usually best tried out first thing in the morning. The more sensitive the eyes, the lower the liver function has become. In Complementary Medicine, the liver and gall bladder also are responsible for the muscles and tendons, therefore when liver chi is under par, muscles are looser, being hurt or pulled more easily and the tendons will be more prone to damage and tearing.

Poor liver and gall bladder function will give rise to headaches and migraines accompanied by a bad temper, because anger is the negative emotion attached to the chi of these organs. (*Refer to* Detox Section).

A Second on the Lips, a Lifetime on the Hips

Besides the obvious superficial attractions of controlling these fatty deposits, there is a more sinister side to cellulite. It is a warning indicating that the liver is over burdened. Therefore this problem needing to be addressed not only for cosmetic purposes but more importantly to improve health and prevent later problems. Sometimes babies are born with a type of cellulite which has been passed on by the mother which can easily be remedied by following this cure, but it will leave the individual more susceptible to cellulite in general.

Even the super models with fat free diets suffer from cellulite. This is due to excess yin food intake such as fruit, salads, drugs, alcohol etc. assisted and aggravated by the intake or excess production of the hormone oestrogen. If one eats simply a yin diet to keep super slim, one will over yinnise the metabolism. This creates an overly yin synthetic state, directing the natural processes of the body to produce more oestrogen. Oestrogen is a hormone which will add fatty tissue to the breasts, hips and thighs etc.. Thus weight will be added to these parts of the anatomy. These areas are, more and more for some women, becoming solely a display of erotic zones. Whereas initially these parts of the body were specific regions displaying instinctual messages to the mate, informing him that they had a healthy potential for offspring. This evolutionary by product was an instinctual method to continue the species, i.e. storage of surplus fat for winter pregnancies, large productive breasts and so forth. This is why these criteria have crept into fashion over the centuries, as people have been able to control their environment more successfully. Thus procreative necessities have evolved into a pleasure principle and eroticism over the centuries.

Hormones

Another source of cellulite causing yin is the synthetic hormone of oestrogen to be found in the female contraceptive pill and pollution in the water supplies from recycled oestrogen. This emanates from various sources such as the contraceptive pill itself, hormones in the food chain used to fatten up livestock as well as oestrogen mimicking substances called xeno-oestrogens. These pollutants originate from agrocides, detergents, plastic bottles, etc.. All having the same effect of yin lateral expansion including depositing fat.

There is a darker side to the unnecessary levels of oestrogens to be found in food and water. They have been linked by many scientists to be a major cause of breast, ovarian, cervical cancers in the female as well as sterility. There is also a link claimed by science that these oestrogens cause impotence and testicular cancer in males. There is also research into the link between oestrogens being responsible for endometriosis. A complaint where the endometrium, the thickened lining of the uterus created during ovulation, can become abnormally displaced throughout the pelvic area during menstruation. This occurs instead of being naturally discharged through the regular channels of menstruation. The waste products can be deposited into the ovaries, causing a lot of pain and discomfort in the abdominal cavity.

Cure

The cure is simple, keep to a vegetarian diet of 70% yang and 30 % yin foods grown naturally in season from 'organic', indigenous sources or from the same climatic zones as you live. This will balance the whole organism, expelling toxins thus easing the liver and gall bladder. The energy or 'chi' of the body will balance itself when the body is functioning normally. More detail can be found how to balance food with the yin yang diet.

The yang should be composed of grains, including millet, cous cous, bulgur, brown rice, barley, corn, oats, rye, buckwheat and buckwheat noodles, and whole grain bread preferably unleavened. Balanced by lightly cooked vegetables such as leeks, chicory, carrots, celery, artichokes, radishes, onions and garlic. Keep seasonal fruit consumption to a minimum. Use only 'virgin' cold pressed oils, olive oil being the most suitable for the liver as well as safflower and sunflower.

Herbs

Herbs which help the liver are, milk thistle, rosemary, thyme, chervil, celery, tarragon, chive, fennel, cumin, capers, nutmeg, clove, horseradish, wild thyme (serpolet), saffron and dandelion. Use herbs as one would a medicine, sparingly and cautiously.

A drink which helps detox the liver and gall bladder is: - hot lemon with pure water slightly sweetened with pure honey first thing before any other drink or food and after meals to help digestion. One can use lemons because of their alkaline effect despite the fact they are citrus fruits and a very yin fruit. However too much lemon juice will over yinnise other parts of the body having undesired results. Therefore avoid taking a lemon cure for more than a month at a time and preferably in the warmer seasons. Other useful aids for the liver are decoctions of, white radish, rosemary, thyme, mint, meadowsweet, and camomile which are also tonifying, (*Refer to* Detox Section).

Avoid dairy foods whenever possible, milk, butter, cheese, eggs, and 'fatty' animal protein and 'oily' fish, and prawns which are very high in cholesterol. All taxing the liver, as will sugar, chocolate, alcohol, chemicals, pharmaceutical medication of all kinds, food additives, colouring and preservatives, cod liver oil, margarine and processed oils, white bread, coffee and milk, vaccines, and foods containing oxalic acid such as tomatoes, spinach and potatoes.

Another useful tip to keep the liver function in good order is to eat foods at the appropriate time. The replenishing chi of the body circulates through the liver and gall bladder from 11.00pm. - 1.00am. & 1.00am - 3.00am. (GMT/Local Solar Time) respectively. Therefore try to retire before these times and eat lightly at least three hours before sleep. Otherwise liver chi is depleted unnecessarily.

Spring is an ideal season for people to detox the liver, around Mardi Gras, as the name implies being 'Fat Tuesday'. Fatty foods which are negative 'liver' foods should be eaten for the last time as Winter closes, then given up until the next cold season. Fats and oils were eaten as a reserve fuel for the winter. Although it is still a sensible time to purge the liver, the types of food are obviously different because these customs evolved prior to supermarkets and central heating. It is not by chance that Mardi Gras coincides with the Complementary Medicine standpoint, when liver energy is revitalised in the yearly cycle around spring.

Exercise and Massage

Massaging the cellulite with oils of rosemary and lavender, all around the area concerned, will improve circulation. Seaweed rubs and sea bathing will also increase circulation. These will increase circulation of blood and chi. It will help to remove fatty deposits, but if the liver is not up to par the fat will stay in the blood and redeposit itself. Therefore one must clean up the system for any relief to be effective for the long term. Even a purge in a health farm will be of little use unless the overall diet is continued to be balanced and relative to liver and gall bladder function.

Sensible exercise is always a tonic for the body and soul. Gentle aerobic exercise, cycling and light jogging will assist burning off stored fatty deposits around the bums and tums.

Exercises like Tai Chi Chuan, Chi Kung and Yoga are excellent for maintaining body balance. Do a variety of standing Chi Kungs from Part 3, such as 1), 3), 4), 7) & 8). Standing Chi Kung will naturally firm up the legs and thighs, increasing circulation naturally as well as burning off fat therefore reducing cellulite. Achieved without forming unsightly muscle, with the added bonus of fortifying all the internal organs and circulatory system without any physical stress. These methods and the dietary guidelines for cellulite are also beneficial for osteoporosis

Always check with a medical practitioner if you are going to take herbal remedies whilst taking prescribed medicines.

Chronic Fatigue Syndrome - ME and Depression

General Symptoms and Causes

CFS or post viral fatigue syndrome, (ME- myalgic encephalomyelitis) is a disorder characterised by around six months or sometimes more of debilitating fatigue that begins suddenly. Including the possible symptoms of a mild fever, sore throat, tender lymph nodes, muscle and joint pains, headache, memory loss, depression and sleep disturbances. The more up to date medical surveys from the United States, have determined that it is mainly focused in young professionals in their mid twenties and thirties, being twice as frequent in women as in men. It tends to follow persistent infection by enteroviruses, with viral material being deposited in the muscles. The virus enters the body through the intestines tending to invade the central nervous system, and depress the immune function. This can result in a post burn out depression of mind and body or sometimes this can simply manifest itself as a general malaise and listlessness. This is usually the result of excess stress on the mind and body.

Exercise can compound the problem by depleting body energy, chi, coupled with reduced muscle tissue oxygen.

Western medicine often states the cause as unknown, simply diagnosing it as possibly emanating from an immune disorder.

The symptoms of CFS point overwhelmingly in favour of a disturbance of the psyche past or present, where drugs can never reach. They only repress the symptoms, not the real reason of the complaint, being a discontent of life itself. Although drugs may give a temporary respite, they have to be weighed up against the long term harmful side effects, which are all too evident. This fact is rarely brought to the attention of the patient by misguided or over worked doctors.

CFS and depression are exacerbated by poor diet usually triggered by a trauma or events leading up to it.

Cure

CFS can be best summed up as chronic 'stress' syndrome, where the mind and its ability to effect the body is just reacting to the soul's need for a change of direction. The problems of life point to a meaning for life. CFS and depression are the result of the inner person, telling the outer person, by way of a shut down, to change lifestyle. The best and most reliable confirmation of such a phenomenon, is generally ignored. This is the inner voice of the eternal experience of the Self, available to all who care to turn on the inner senses. The Self is the centre of one's being which usually communicates to one's outer personality by way of dreams. Therefore one needs to 'turn off, to turn on', by dimming the sole focus of one's attention away from the outside world. Then the inner wisdom can surface into the psyche, with all its eternal help and advice. This tried and tested formula, besides bringing to the fore the path of self-knowledge, will start an exciting adventure into the meaning of life itself. It is the much sought after philosopher's stone. So CFS is actually the psyche's way of guiding a person to a meaningful existence. This look at one's life should be coupled with a balanced diet for an all round cure. (*See* Yin Yang Diet in Part 1). Herbs that can help the cure are

Echinacea which enhances the immune function but should only be taken for two to three weeks as it is yin substance. Sensible amounts of garlic in the diet will boost the immune system, as will ginkgo biloba and good quality ginseng which will also yangise and strengthen the organism.

Tension Creates Growth

This existing approach to the depression of CFS now turns into a welcome bonus, because the natural dimming of the projecting light of the ego, is directed away, in part from the outer chaos of life. Thus allowing the ego to act as a reflecting mirror of one's own inner nature which is the gateway to the collective unconscious. This is usually initiated by dreams but with practice one can develop a form of meditation Carl Jung called, active imagination. Active imagination is where one reflects inwardly, summoning up the wisdom of the collective unconscious. This can take the form of spontaneous thoughts and hunches that seem to come from nowhere, even in extreme cases visions that can appear all too real. But inner voices must be carefully analysed to differentiate between potential destructive fantasies of suppressed complexes as opposed to valid information from the unconscious. (*See* Stress Section or for more detail my book ***Time for a Change.***

The safest place to start is by acknowledging dreams and trying to discover their underlying message. Just as with any subject, continued effort will improve the skill. However do not buy a book of dream interpretation as they tend to dictate dogmatic precepts which are inaccurate as each person is different. The meaning of a dream is portrayed by its own personal symbolism, although the format is archetypal. Always write down or even draw the contents in a diary. Dreams are a compensation for outer life creating a balanced whole. Try to interpret them Jung style, rather like decoding the metaphorical meaning buried in a myth, legend or the all too real significance of the apparent absurdity of a fairy tale.

Femme Fatale and Bluebeard

For example if a man dreams of a Rapunzel type figure, the young girl in a fairy tale who is imprisoned in a tower. Instead of this being a male fantasy of imprisoning women, it is more likely to be a symbol of his feminine side and his feelings, being locked up inside. This can make a man become a slave to his career at the expense of a natural relationship to partners or Mother Nature herself. Both being destructive.

For example women can sometimes dream of a menacing 'bluebeard' type of character, who wants to do them harm. This frightening figure of her psyche might attract her, albeit unconsciously, to men with malevolent agendas. This male side to a woman's personality, if left in the dark, can drive a female to pursue a goal which can violate her femininity. Hence the dream of a threatening male figure or beast.

This dark unconscious side to the personality of both women and men is destructive to relationships and life. When these discarded parts of the soul are integrated into consciousness, their negative unconscious power is abated. Jung stated that we meet our unconscious as fate, because we project our unconscious out into the world, until it is truly and honestly reflected by the individual.

This is and was the role of rituals in all cultures as rites if suitably engaged in, would draw down the barrier between the conscious and unconscious aspects of the psyche. These inner aspects of our soul, when transformed become inner guides of truth. This is the true role of dreams which Dr. Jung proved time and time again. Dreams are an objective voice of inner truth. For a detailed discussion of this empirical phenomenon, please refer to the relevant sections from Jung's collected works or the books of Dr. Marie-Louise Von Franz, on how to correctly interpret dreams.

Now the symptoms of CFS and depression mature into a failsafe. The organism shuts down in order to realign itself, being in reality a path of enlightenment. Therefore CFS or depression can be turned into a positive happening to improve and give meaning to one's life, thus every cloud has a silver lining.

Besides a general sea change, a healthy diet will speed up recovery. The balanced diet in this book will harmonise the mind and body as well as making a statement of intent to improve the situation. Particular attention is needed to avoid foods with chemicals additives and preservatives, because they yinnise or slow down the mental faculties. In the same way as alcohol and all types of drugs whether recreational or prescribed. Therefore try and avoid drugs, alcohol and stimulants until well on the way to recovery. In Germany doctors have successfully revived the use of St. John's Wort, hypericum, as a nervine that is a herb that calms the organism, relieving migraines and neuralgia as well.

Exercise

Tai Chi and Chi Kung are excellent at strengthening internal energy and confidence, in a carefully controlled manner. These types of disciplines accompanied by a balanced diet and reflection will fortify the mind and the body allowing the metamorphosis to take place smoothly.

If there are no suitable Tai Chi teachers or it is not convenient to learn and practice these exercises, one can take walks or breaks, far from the madding crowd. Always in natural environments amongst friends, allowing the simplicity of mother nature to permeate, thus supporting the healing process. Despite the temporary attractions of lively places full of people having a good time, they should be avoided when feeling low, as they offer a very synthetic recess. Fun places are forms of collective escapism which although offering a temporary respite, can actually increase depression. One can never run from oneself.

This natural approach has a deep healing potential, permitting the mind and body to centre themselves, returning the senses to a normal state. Healing can only take place if one is relaxed and tranquil which is helped by listening to pleasant music and reading inspirational books.

The suggested Chi Kungs from Part 3 will help build up the immune system as well generally toning up the mind and body being 1), 1a), 2), 8) & 9). They are helpful and healing, but please make sure to read the introductory passages from the Part 3, on Chi Kung as well.

Always check with a medical practitioner if you are going to take herbal remedies whilst taking prescribed medicines.

Colds and Flu

Common Colds

Common Colds and flu, although different, are caused by excesses of yin and yang foods as well as lifestyle. Cold symptoms are usually red itching eyes, clear nasal discharge progressing to yellow and thick, mild sore throat, and low fever, blocked nose and a cough. A cold is usually caused by an excess diet of yin or yang, especially industrialised foodstuffs like burgers, soft drinks, fruit and salads out of season, dairy food, alcohol, as well as over consumption of potatoes, tomatoes, bananas, citrus and tropical fruit and spices etc.. The cold is the body's seasonal way of expelling toxins, so must be allowed to run its natural course otherwise toxins are retained in the body. This is more likely to happen around the spring and autumn solstices in March and September as the weather changes. An excess of yin and or yang food and drink in winter will be expelled in spring. The same occurs if an excess is consumed in summer, nature will naturally try and throw off the residues in autumn preparing one's organism for winter. This phenomenon occurs more and more now with the global village when one travels rapidly between climates and seasons. Also colds can be a reaction to stress or a trauma making the body clear out and rest.

Nevertheless do not take medicines that suppress the symptoms even though conveniently available from pharmacies. This will only delay the onset of more serious manifestations at a later date besides reducing the natural immune function. Also stay clear of prescribed anti-biotics as these will also weaken the body's natural defence mechanism. Symptomatic cures can weaken the organism giving a window for more serious illnesses later. Therefore do not be alarmed by the discharge of mucous from the nose, sinuses and lungs as this a healthy clear out, just see it through.

Influenza or Flu

Influenza or flu is a contagious infection, usually of the lungs, caused by a virus and transmitted by airborne particles. It occurs in isolated cases and as epidemics. The symptoms are more acute than a common cold including sore throat, cough, fever, aching muscles and joints, and general weakness. Higher fever and non-local symptoms distinguish influenza from the common cold. The incubation period is short around 1-3 days. The onset is usually sudden, with chills, fever, and general malaise. The various flu viruses attack those with a weaker immune function due to poor diet, persistent use of anti-biotics, chaotic lifestyle and sometimes over exercise. The elderly and young are particularly at risk; therefore as prevention is better than cure, ensure a balanced diet and lifestyle in order to prevent illness and try to avoid vaccinations. The balanced diet in this book will ensure a natural self-defence system against disease. One can expect flu to be cleared, depending on the severity and the person in anything from 3-10 days.

Cure

Plenty of rest and quiet in friendly natural surroundings. Try and stay out of bed as this will reduce symptoms, but do not be over active as this uses up vital energy needed for healing. Stay warm at all times. Occasional baths with essential oils like peppermint and rosemary will increase circulation thus speed up recovery by helping to expel toxins.

To aid the cleansing process, teas made from elderflower, peppermint, catmint, feverfew, natural liquorice and St. John's Wort are efficacious. A tried and tested expectorant is essence of cinnamon. Inhalation of Friar's balsam and or Olbas Oil are also useful to clear lungs and sinuses.

Therefore whilst recovering avoid all extremes of yin and yang foods. (*See* Yin Yang Diet) Drink plenty of clean, pure liquids and for sustenance have broths and soups made from organic grain and vegetable sources avoiding potatoes, tomatoes and fruit. Echinacea and garlic capsules will help boost the immune function as well as acting as a natural anti-biotic.

Exercise

Avoid any stressful or strenuous exercise, but one can do seated or lying down Chi Kungs 1 & 2 from Part 3. Whilst recovering, basic Tai Chi Chuan and Yoga will help clear the breathing as well as strengthening the internal organs, ease aching muscles and limbs, and will help focus the mind and spirit. Best if carried out early morning.

Always check with a medical practitioner if you are going to take herbal remedies whilst taking prescribed medicines.

'Detoxing'

'Detoxing', although in reality is not an actual word, is becoming a household term for undoing that which modern society does to itself. This expression would not exist if there were no toxins. Therefore by its very existence one accepts that toxins are absorbed on a daily basis. However the best cure is always prevention, so it is far wiser to be constantly alert in order to minimise toxin intake from food, air, water and the environment. These factors have been covered in my yin yang diet, however human nature, from time to time needs more than bread alone. Therefore after any overindulgence, one should always centre the diet in harmony with the season and climate as per the yin yang diet. This encourages the body's natural ability to purge itself. It is useful to have some natural substances, to hand, that will help the cleansing process, these with dietary hints and the deep breathing exercises at the end of this section. Detoxing, superficially seems a new idea, but is connected to past rituals of purification.

Fasting

The historical ancestor of detoxing, is fasting. The connection between the two, even though not openly apparent, is because all things in the present are built upon the past, just as our back leg is the impetus for forward movement. The modern cleansing, albeit for health reasons, has its roots in the tradition of ritual fasting which has been recorded since antiquity in cultures from all over the world. The general idea being to purify the body to become more receptive to the inner experience, enabling one to cope with the outside world in a more balanced fashion. Whereas present day detoxing is considered a method to support health so as to do battle more effectively against the outer pressures, it has in effect, the same goal, albeit in a different guise. Because the outer world is a mere projection of the inner one, both cleansing processes are ways to refresh the organism in a form of self-sacrifice, with both producing the desired effect by self-discipline.

Witch Doctors

The Shamans of the Indians from the Great Plains of North America would fast, as well as using a sweat lodge to cleanse the mind and body in order that the tribe could seek out and hunt the wild game more effectively, thus ensuring the survival of the tribe. The shamans of the Inuit in the frozen wastelands sharpened their senses by fasting and inner cleansing, for the same vital reasons of endurance. The Greeks of the Hellenistic world had several rites of fasting such as the dedicated practice of not eating before one could receive the cure which would then be transmitted as a dream or vision in the Temple dedicated to Ascelepius, a father of Western medicine. The Pythagoreans, besides being famous for the geometry, were a devoted numerological cult also using fasting as a method of receiving divine inspiration from the gods, including their calculus. The mystical cult of Orpheus, a sacrificial God of Ancient Greece was a precursor to Christianity. The Orphic rites were based on the solar calendar of the zodiac, the twelve Christian Apostles equating to the twelve signs of the zodiac with the thirteenth one, acting as a solar Deity of reconciliation. In both cases being a sacrificial act, taking the form of a ritual death giving rise to an annual renewal or rebirth, in accordance with the seasons. The Orphic doctrine had many sacrificial rituals of purification in order to enhance the inner person by cleansing the outer shell. Christianity also absorbed and rearranged many Middle Eastern traditions which included ritual fasting from the Jewish calendar, such as Yom Kippur, the Day of Atonement. This transformed into the penitence of the forty days of fasting of Lent before Easter, besides Ash Wednesday, Good Friday, Advent and so forth. Islam has the month of Ramadan where the Muslims deny themselves all sustenance during the hours of light in an act of faith to their Creator. The modern difference between the dates is because the Jewish and Muslim calendar is based on the cycles of the moon which loops in and out of the solar cycle which predominates in Christianity. The Hindu mystics also abstained from eating in order to become closer to the, Atman, the cosmic Self. In China, there was a ritual fasting and abstinence during the night of the winter solstice (21st December). This sacred rite celebrated the birth of the Heavenly Yang energy which began the following day, accompanied by the inevitable increase of daylight. The Taoists would cleanse their systems by living purely on meditative chi for extensive periods, with mysterious legends of adepts surviving without food at all, in order to allow their inner chi to vibrate at the same pitch as the cosmic chi of the Tao.

Affluence and Toxins

Today's detoxing in the first world is a cyclical consequence, derived from the excesses of Western living. Human nature being what it is, has given rise to the compensatory abundance of foodstuffs. This is only a human compensation, to make up for the collective deprivation of food from the past. Unfortunately this surplus, is poor quality nutrition, being supplied by factory farming with all its hidden dangers. Although our wealthy forbears did not go hungry, they eat an overly rich diet, predominantly a surfeit of animal protein supplemented with negligible amounts of grains and fresh vegetables. These practices were not based on nutrition, but the fact that animal foodstuffs were a symbol of their wealth and power. This was also a symbol of dominance, symbolically raising affluent humans above the considered chaos of the animal kingdom. Whereas the poor were obliged to eat a humble diet in squalid conditions. Both suffered through their lack of consciousness.

Now it is ironic that the first world has banished basic malnutrition and the 'old' diseases, only to replace them with new dangers from new diseases like cancer exacerbated by pollution, industrialised foods and super bugs. Generally, the third world and indigenous peoples had more balanced diets due to the smaller, more traditional groups where tried and tested methods were handed down through the tight knit communities. This was conditioned by the extreme climates of the frozen north or the fierce weather and diseases of the tropics. These conditions prevented the less inventive husbandry and food cultivation of the safer, more predictable and controllable temperate zones of Europe. Unfortunately both good and bad techniques have now migrated to all corners of the world.

Sacrifice

In effect present day detoxing is a form of sacrifice. This word is derived from the Latin, 'sacrificus', sacer-sacred, holy + ficus-facere, to make', in other words to 'sacred make' or make sacred, whole (holy) or balanced. This sort of sacrifice or denial has always been a necessary clearing out of the body's toxins and demons. Generally it is and was easier to perform these cleansing principles when people were bound to collective rituals. This is now much more difficult because of the present, contrary collective focus of self-interest consumerism. Even nowadays, with the advent of the media bombardment of all the wonder cures, it is becoming clearer by the day to many people that all these panaceas and so called scientific advances do not live not up to the projected expectations. Notwithstanding the considerable efforts of the 'capital rich' and their vested interests who peddle these new wonder cures and false dreams. Of course these media illusions can never be fulfilled, because life and history prove that one cannot cheat the forces of nature.

There is an old Chinese proverb that one should only pay one's doctor when well. Alas no one has ever outwitted or beaten the natural forces for long which the Chinese codified as complimentary and antagonistic energy levels calling the two relative potentials, of yin and yang. So if we err temporarily from a balanced regime, it is fairly easy, with a little self-discipline, to correct the excesses and harmonise the internal energy back to normal.

Time for a Detox

Therefore in order to detox in a sensible manner it is advisable to follow a balanced diet which will not only realign weight but also allow the body to harmonise itself naturally. There are many detox diets which can be counter productive because they do not follow the principles of yin and yang. For example, people often go on 'fruit, salad or raw food diets' which will cleanse the body to a degree, but rarely are the chemical pesticides, fertilisers etc. considered. These pernicious toxins are held in the skins of the fruit, salad or vegetable, as well as being readily absorbed into the flesh of the foodstuff itself. Therefore, even though, there maybe a weight loss and some relative cleansing achieved, the concentration of other dangerous toxins will be assimilated by the body. Also 'faddy' diets do not take into consideration the yin yang clock of the seasons or the climate. I often come across cases of people being ill in spring as they have gone on a fruit cleansing diet after the excesses of Christmas. This is because they have made the body cold and weak by eating cold food as well as the toxins. This reduces the immune function with a knock on effect to the next energy season, being in this case spring. These unbalanced regimes will do more harm in the long term damaging the immune function and the circulatory system. Leaving the body feeling the cold much more, as well as adversely affecting the muscles, tendons, and the skeletal structure. This overall yinnisation of organism will also yinnise or slow down, both the mind and body.

Chi and Toxins

Modern science is coming to terms with the fact that the body has an independent energy field and circadian rhythm which the Chinese Masters discovered and codified some four and a half thousand years ago. These Masters understood the body to have an inner energy, which they called chi with its two aspects (*See* Yin Yang Diet and Chi Kung Sections). The contracting pitch is described as being yin, counterbalanced by its expanding phase of yang. These two forces are recognised in various forms by many cultures and sciences, albeit with different titles. However the Chinese culture retained this information in tact due to the fact that it is the only continuous uninterrupted civilisation.

This is also reinforced by the need to cope with always having had a relatively large population, living in a huge country with a great variety of terrain and climate. This created their unparalleled system of internal medicine. Wholly based on the principle of the variety of energetic forces emanating from the Universe. The collective title, they gave this life force or 'breath', was chi, which is in either a relative yang or yin state. (*Refer* to Part 3 for a description of chi).

The yin yang diet allows the body to realign the chi into an harmonious condition, strengthening the internal organs which in turn will cause the body to reject all the excesses and unnatural substances whether they are toxins, mucous, fatty substances, pathogens etc.. When the chi is flowing naturally and uninhibited, it will balance the organism into homeostasis.

Inner Cleansing

The main organs of elimination are firstly, the bowels which are fortified and stimulated by whole grains especially organic brown rice which contains phytin acid. This substance helps expel toxins as well as being the most digestible of all the grains with the highest content of the B vitamins which also cleanse the digestive tract. Organic brown rice or barley 'Miso' paste in soups or with vegetables is an excellent way of clearing the digestive system. Irrevocable proof of its detoxifying qualities were field tested by George Oshawa in his clinic outside Nagasaki, when the US airforce dropped their second atomic bomb on Japan in 1946. His patients drank natural miso soup every morning, and even though recovering from other illnesses, were not affected by the nuclear fallout.

Secondly the kidneys perform their tireless work more efficiently when 'dry', in other words one should attempt to keep pure clean liquid intake to c. ¾ - 1 litre a day depending on activity. If the kidneys have to filter large amounts of fluid out of the system they become 'water logged' so their cleansing 'sponge like' action is impaired as well as being an unnecessary burden on these hard working organs. A saturated sponge cannot clean or absorb properly nor can water logged kidneys. The current medical opinion to drink voluminous quantities of liquid derives from the need to water down the toxins from the over processed food and drink, which in the long term is counter productive.

Also the kidneys are adversely effected by too much yang in the form of animal protein especially red meat, eggs, dairy food, salt and its by products including the 'savoury' food additives such as monosodium glutamate and chemical food preservatives to be found in prepared meats.

The liver works in tandem with the kidney and when one of them is under stress, the other will be less effectual. Last but not least, liver function is disturbed by excess yin in the form of sugar, especially white sugar and its by products in jams and soft drinks etc., artificial sweeteners, chemicals, yin drugs, alcohol, spices and tropical fruits etc.. Therefore these complicated foods with their hidden substances, must be reduced or eliminated for successful detoxing. A stressed liver cannot carry out its necessary functions of cleansing the blood and the some sixty or so other major biological functions. When this organ is overburdened it can adversely effect its production of cholesterol which forms arteriosclerosis, clogged arteries which can cause heart disease and strokes etc..

Liver Test

A simple test to check liver and gall bladder function is the performance of their associated sense organs of the eyes. If the eyes are losing focus or over sensitive to sunlight early in the morning or bright lights at night, the chi of the liver is under par. The left shoulder is sometimes higher than the right, caused by an overburdened and enlarged liver which is situated in the opposite energy and physical zone of the torso, under the lower right ribcage.

The lungs are also main stream organs of elimination which are strained by pollution as well as from tobacco smoke and poor quality air, reducing their ability to expel carbon dioxide in turn effecting visceral efficiency. The lungs in Complementary Medicine effect the body hair and skin which is the largest organ of the body also acting as a medium of toxin elimination. For example psoriasis is where the toxins are at such an overload that the skin is used to displace the excess toxicity. This is usually generated by too much liquid, normally poor quality alcohol or soft drinks and too much animal protein, catalysed by smoking and polluted air. (*See* Skin Trouble in this section).

Lungs and Skin

Skin trouble is often accompanied by lung complaints. When the lungs are in good order, its brother organ of the large intestine will perform its major role of elimination unhindered. Air baths and exposing the skin to the air for sensible periods without catching cold, are ways to help its major role in 'breathing' for the body. The body loses several pounds of skin in its lifetime and is the main constituent of house dust. The skin is constantly adjusting itself to temperature by opening and closing the pores to help maintain a constant temperature and homeostasis. One obvious biological function is its ability to dispel fluid by sweat in order to cool and cleanse. This phenomenon is exploited in saunas and steam baths etc. which are a proven aid to body and tissue purification, which must not be excessive, due to the potential of excessive fluid and mineral loss.

It is obvious that the body works at its natural optimum, when all the component parts are inter acting correctly. The following procedures will assist nature to rebalance the internal energy and the organs thus promote detoxification, whilst adopting the yin yang dietary procedures.

The lungs need plenty of fresh clean air, enhanced by deep breathing especially, reverse breathing, (*See* Part 3). The eliminating action of the bowel works at its optimum on a diet of well chewed natural whole grains and vegetables. The bowel does not perform as well if it has to extract large irregular amount of liquid from its domain, however pure.

Colonic Irrigation

This is best avoided as it will reduce the natural action of the food.

Detox Herbs for the Kidney

The filtering of the kidneys are assisted by the herbs and plants of: - fennel, parsley, chervil, tarragon, sage, burdock, bladderwort, dandelion and nettle. The latter four acting as natural diuretics which can be drunk as infusions. White radish can be eaten peeled and grated (like carrots) in salads or made into an decoction i.e. c. 8oz. of peeled grated white radish simmered in a pint of filtered water reduced by 1/3rd, helps detox the liver as well as acting as a diuretic. This vegetable is effective at reducing the results of eating too much dairy food and animal protein.

Good quality ginseng, in small regular doses, will strengthen kidney function for men whereas women should take ginseng in a medium such as Royal Gelée, otherwise it can over yangise the female chi. A simple guide to see if kidney chi is up to par is that the natural desire for sex is improved and enhanced. There should also be a regular ability to pass fluids which should be a clear golden colour. The colour of the urine could darken and smell unpleasant whilst displacing toxins, but this should only be a temporary situation for a relatively healthy person who does not have any serious problems. A persistent dark urine can indicate an organ dysfunction which needs medical diagnosis. (*See* Digestive Disorders in this section). Also during or just after a detox the faeces can be dark and hard or the other extreme of being pale and loose. This can be normal at this time but must not persist more than a week. If so medical attention is needed.

Daily Detox Exercise

A general massage and Chi Kung for the kidneys and their essence (pre-birth chi) are as follows: -

First thing after rising in the morning, drink an infusion of one of the four natural diuretics (*See above*) then :-

1) Rub the ears gently forwards and backwards with the fingers, this will help wake up the kidneys and their chi in the morning.

2) Rub, in a stroking motion, both hands down the outside (yang) of the legs and then back up towards the body on the inside (yin) of the legs, then with one hand, rub in a stroking motion outward away from the body along the outside of the arm (yang) and back up towards the body on the inside of the arm.

3) Gently tap the lower back over the kidney area with lightly clenched fists being very beneficial in stimulating the internal energy of the 'kidney'. K1, an acupoint, at the centre of the pad of the feet can be stimulated by hand massage etc. or even with a lighted moxa herb bundle or even an incense stick.

Detox Herbs for the Liver

Herbs which help the liver are :- rosemary, thyme, chervil, celery, tarragon, chive, fennel, cumin, capers, nutmeg, clove, horseradish, wild thyme (serpolet), saffron and dandelion.

'Real' liquorice, that has little or no sugar in a natural a state as is possible, is an excellent tonic for the liver and helps clear out toxins. Milk thistle, artichoke extract and echinacea are herbal preparations that can be bought in most health food shops, being excellent herbs that tone the liver function, as well as promoting the removal of toxins.

Drinks which help detox the liver and gall bladder are:- hot lemon and pure water slightly sweetened with pure honey first thing before any other drink or food and after meals to help digestion. Lemon juice although becoming an alkali in the stomach, is still very yin therefore must be used carefully especially in cold weather or seasons and should be stopped if the body becomes prone to cold, circulation is reduced, chestiness, lethargy, headaches, tiredness or if any other 'yin' symptoms prevail. Decoctions of rosemary, thyme, mint, meadowsweet, and camomile are also excellent tonics for the liver. Use only for a week at a time.

Herbs including lemon juice should be treated as one would a medicine with caution and respect.

Chi Kungs, from Part 3 which help detox the body and reinforce the internal organs are:- 1), 2), 6), 7) & 8) which will have the best results if carried out early morning.

Finally to sum up, the best way to detox whether long term or short term is to do it gradually as a sudden detoxification can be a shock to the system. If one fasts away from food, clean liquid is a must so as to keep the kidney clean otherwise kidney stones can form. Fasting or detoxing can result in the body discharging in the form of 'colds', loose bowel movement, unusual amounts and colour of urine and faecal evacuation, spots, mucous discharge from lungs or sinuses. As a result of the cleansing process one can undergo, temporary symptoms of a cold or a chill with a mild temperature during the detox. This is a natural side effect, when the body is expelling the surfeit of yin and yang energy that has become locked in the organism. When going through a cleansing process try to consume more food before midday and less or none afterwards.

Tai Chi, Chi Kung and Exercise

Another aid to detoxing is to do sensible amounts of non-strenuous exercise, like Tai Chi Chuan, Chi Kung, Yoga, walking, sea bathing, cycling, leisure tennis and so forth. All of these preferably carried out in natural environments, in conjunction with wholesome food based on the principles of the yin yang diet in this book, but always carried out in a careful manner.

A sensible balanced programme of detoxification as outlined above, will not only clear the organism resulting in a brighter fresher mind and body but can return the natural weight and shape to the disciplined individual. This will allow one to deal with the inevitable adversities of one's daily pursuits in a more centred and unruffled fashion.

Always check with a medical practitioner if you are going to take herbal remedies whilst taking prescribed medicines.

Diabetes

General Symptoms and Causes

Diabetes Milletus is a hybrid word comprised of the Greek word, diabainein, 'to pass through' and the Latin, mellitus 'sweetened with honey'. It has been recognized as a disease since antiquity. Probably so named because of the amount of honey or sweetness consumed. The ancient world of Arcadia around the Mediterranean consumed excess amounts of honey, as it was considered a nectar associated with deification. Probably supplemented by the many various euphoric, alcoholic by-products made from or sweetened with honey. This over consumption of yin food and drink resulted in the subsequent passing through of the excess sweetness into the urinary bladder which linked our forbears with the all too familiar criteria of modern diabetes.

Diabetes Milletus is caused by the failure of the islets of Langherhans to produce enough insulin. The hyposecretion of insulin, being a yang hormone, results in an overly yin blood condition. Where the sugar level in the blood rises, causing hyperglycemia with symptoms of thirst, tiredness, loss of weight accompanied by the unpleasant, excessive production of urine. The symptomatic signs of diabetes initially manifest themselves as tiredness and fatigue as the sugar levels rise above 130 mg per decilitre (100cc) of blood. If it continues to rise above 180 mg, it approaches the renal threshold. At this point, the tubules of the kidneys are unable to reabsorb all of the glucose filtered by the glomeruli, being the main filtering structure of the kidneys. This causes sugar to appear in the urine, glycosuria, needing more water to discharge the excess glucose thus increasing the urine discharge to abnormal levels which is called, polyuria. This loss of water in diabetics causes the unusual thirst, accompanied by the loss of glucose and minerals inducing a ravenous appetite. Diabetes adversely interferes with the metabolism of sugar and the oxidation of fats, which in turn is dependent on the oxidation of glucose, also being disrupted. The partially oxidised fats give rise to ketone bodies and acetone which also appear in the urine. Sometimes causing the smell of acetone on the breath. When these and other acidic ketones are in profusion, it leaches the body's mineral reserves because of the acidosis, preventing efficient carbon dioxide discharge. The carbon dioxide and the acidosis become toxic elements for the body, resulting in possible convulsions, diabetic coma and even death.

Yin and Diabetes

High blood sugar being very yin, seriously effects the circulation, reducing blood flow to the peripheral parts of the body, especially the lower limbs and feet as well as the hands. This condition also reduces skin elasticity, preventing wounds healing normally, also ulcers can develop. Diabetes can harm the teeth due to the mineral loss caused by this disease. It also weakens the eye sight due to the yinnisation of the internal energy of the eye, as well as the damage to the retina, retinopathy. The section on improving eye sight and visual function can improve the impaired vision caused by diabetes.

Type 1 Diabetes

There are two classes of diabetes; Type 1, known as 'Insulin Dependent' which is to be found more commonly in children or adolescents which is harder to cure as they are born or contract it early in life and have become 'Insulin Dependent'. This is where the diabetic is unable to produce sufficient insulin being the hormone that transports glucose, a simple sugar, into the cells of the body for fuel. Normally due to a very yin constitution which may have been caused by DNA mutation before or during pregnancy coupled with over yin consumption and chaotic eating by parents.

Type 2 Diabetes

Type 2, 'Non Insulin Dependent', normally occurs at the onset of middle age and or obesity, which is less severe and easier to cure. This is where there is enough insulin in the body but the person is unable to absorb the glucose into the cell despite the presence of insulin. This is where the person has become very yang, i.e. often overweight due to consumption of industrialised foods especially excess sugar and fatty substances with lack of exercise.

Yin and Yang and Diabetes

If one applies the logic of yin and yang, it is quite easy to categorise the cause of diabetes and put forward a balancing remedy. The extent of the cure will depend on the long term damage to the internal organs concerned. In a normal person insulin is secreted in the pancreas by the islets of Langerhans. The masses of these cells are focused around the tail end of the pancreas. The more yang beta cells within the islets secrete insulin, whilst the larger yin alpha cells produce glucagon. In diabetes the yang beta cells become expanded or yinnised, losing their ability to produce insulin. This yinnisation is caused by an overly yin blood condition, usually as a result of consuming too much industrialised foods containing amongst other yin substances, sugar and sugar by-products, fruit and spices. This is exacerbated by eating foods out of season and climate as well as exposure to the modern yin chemicals and pollutants. Also dairy food and heavy animal protein contribute to this over yin or acidic condition. Owing to the genetic differentials of people, different foods will have relative consequences on different people, but in general terms, individuals with a pancreatic weakness can become diabetic because of high acidity from foodstuffs creating this yin condition.

People who have had organ transplants are similarly affected by the anti-rejection drugs, which after a period, can contract a drug induced Type 2 diabetes, for the same yin reasons. Even in these more extreme cases, the diabetes can be assisted considerably by balancing diet and lifestyle.

It is also considered that both types of diabetes are linked to the loss of auto-immunity, because diabetics produces antibodies that destroy their own beta cells. This auto-immunity is also caused by the over yinnisation or dilation of the internal energy of the body which is the power behind the immune system. Yang energy is responsible for the protective aspect of the immune function. Whereas yin energy of the organism is the attacking aspect.

Cure

The accepted medical procedure for Diabetes is to inject insulin directly into the bloodstream, this has an instant effect of stabilising the blood sugar and has saved many lives, but as diabetes is an extreme yin blood condition, it really needs a diet with a natural yang emphasis. Being ever mindful not to over yangise the system because this can cause the all too human weakness, to swing to the other extreme, resulting in an over compensating indulgence in yin foodstuffs. The yangisation can take place, without any harm, whilst the diabetic is taking insulin, adjusting the dose relative to the ability of the pancreas to produce insulin.

Research published 2002 at Harvard University Boston, USA has shown that diet plays an important part in controlling Type 1 Diabetes and curing Type 2 diabetes. The studies indicating a vegan diet with an emphasis on whole grains, are deemed to be the best. Inspired by this tried and tested yin yang system of healing.

Type 2 Diabetes can be Cured

Type 2 can be completely cured if a balanced diet and appropriate exercise are adhered to. Type 1 can also be better controlled and healed if the diabetic strictly follows the yin yang diet, accompanied by a general balanced regime. However this is more difficult needing greater will power and self control, but still possible because the cells of the pancreas, especially in the young can regenerate. If the cure is not complete, the diabetes can certainly be ameliorated and controlled by applying the yin yang principles. Supplemented, if necessary by the prescribed insulin, but with less dependence. The time and effort of the cure will depend on the damage to the pancreas caused by the inherited genetic defects and or the length of time of insulin dependence.

The Pancreas and Diabetes

Diabetes is the inability of the pancreas to produce enough 'yang' insulin by way of the islets of Langherhans, normally brought about by an excess consumption of sugar and sugar products like jam, soft drinks etc., fruit, dairy food like butter, milk, cheese and eggs, junk foods with chemicals, spices consumed in the wrong climate, the varied cocktail of preservatives and colouring etc., excess animal protein, especially poor quality 'factory farmed' meat and most forms of drugs. Exacerbated by the ever increasing stress of modern life and the continuing onslaught of pollution from the air, water supplies and food (*See* Part 1). This over yin eating can be a family trait, or people eating foods that are not compatible with the climate. Diabetes can start in the womb caused by a pregnant mother's over indulgence of the above yin foods. These will disturb the cell structure of the pancreas belonging to the innocent, yet dependent child that she is carrying.

Diet and Diabetes

Therefore the body must be carefully yangised, by centering the diet, ensuring to avoid all the yin foods, especially all industrialized foods. As well as yin environments that are damp

or polluted by toxins or electro-magnetic fields. To create the right conditions for a full or partial cure from diabetes, one must adopt the general guidelines from the yin yang diet, with an emphasis on the following foods and proportions:-
50%-60% bias of yang type whole organic cereal grains should be consumed, especially short grain brown rice, barley, millet and buckwheat. All containing essential B vitamins, particularly millet. They serve as a catalyst to produce various hormones, including insulin.

20%-30% of the diet should consist of yang, naturally grown vegetables, especially the root varieties of carrots, turnips, swede, as well as leeks, onion and the firmer greens including cabbage, cauliflower, brussel sprouts, green beans etc.. All preferably cooked in a yang fashion, that is boiled in little water or baked, preferably without oil or fat.

Try and eat more oven cooked food in colder weather, as opposed to faster cooking during milder climates such as stir frying. Always using small amounts of good quality, organic cold pressed virgin oils, or preferably sesame or corn oil. A tip to ensure that vegetables remain crisp, tastily nutritious and not over yinnised, is that they should be cooked quickly, in a limited amount of water, adding a little oil to prevent burning. This reduces all the water with the oil sealing the vegetable, acting like a built in steamer, thus conserving all the vital nutrients. Remember oil and fat encourage Type 2 Diabetes so use oil sparingly.

Taboos

Diabetics should avoid potatoes, spinach, tomatoes, aubergine, rhubarb, bananas, mangos, egg plants, ketchup, spicy sauces etc. and all the yin tropical fruit and vegetables. Unless they live in the tropics, but also then kept to a minimum in hot climates.

Use salt sparingly, preferably seasoning with good quality organic soya sauce and sesame salt (*See* Yin Yang Diet).

10%-15% small yang type pulses and beans like lentils are especially beneficial for diabetics. Avoiding the yin chick pea if possible.

5% inclusion of seaweed in the diet is an excellent source of minerals and vitamins. Seaweed is now more popular and available, but as always be vigilant of its source due to the ever increasing rate of sea pollution.

The ever healing garlic, in moderation, is helpful in diabetes as it boosts the immune system as well as helping to remove glucose from the blood.

Liquid

Liquid must be kept pure, simple and limited to c. ½-¾ of a litre depending on activity, avoiding regular coffee, tea and alcohol, soft drinks especially the 'sugar free' variety as most sugar substitutes are more harmful than the sugar they replace. Good quality ginseng can be very beneficial for Type 1 Diabetes as well. Other herbs that are helpful for diabetics are fenugreek, goat's rue, gentian, burdock and elderflower, the latter two being generally available as herbal teas whereas the former are available as preparations in health food stores.

Cooking and Chewing

Never cook in a microwave as the food, although technically cooked, is harmfully yinnised due to the radiation of high-frequency electromagnetic waves.

Diabetics must chew food thoroughly, eating smaller quantities of food more often. Never eating late in the evening, allowing several hours of any light meal to be well digested before retiring.

Besides the appropriate exercise if one wants to attempt a complete cure the above dietary suggestions should be strictly adhered to, long after the symptoms abate. The insulin must always be continued, but one can adjust the amount as one feels better. This process of self-empowerment will add to the healing process, even though a complete cure may not be achieved. But one will be more in charge of one's destiny and less dependent. Always bearing in mind that there will be a potential weakness in the pancreas which must be respected.

Although these measures may seem difficult, weighed up against the long term effects of diabetes they are well worth the investment. Thus preventing high blood pressure, heart disease, asthma, kidney problems and eye disorders. These measures will initiate more freedom, self control and even a complete cure of diabetes.

Why?

If a diabetic is attempting to heal him or herself in this way, a time of reflection and consultation with the inner voice of wisdom is suggested. This open self analysis can lead to a profound understanding of life, by asking such questions; 'Why did it happen to me ?'; 'Do I really want to be cured ?'; 'Who is to blame, humankind or God?,' and so forth. I have often found that an affliction of any kind, major or minor if accepted can pave the way to a life with real meaning. This can have considerable healing qualities for the soul as well as the body. The solution always lies at the centre of the problem.

On a more practical note, the diabetic should adjust his or her insulin levels, after about a month of the controlled eating, the change in outlook and lifestyle. Thereafter judging and carefully administering the amount of insulin on a quid pro quo basis, depending on the quality of the diet, environment, level of exercise, feeling of well being, self confidence etc.. Maybe with enough will power one can notably relieve and even cure the diabetes.

Exercise and Massage

A diabetic should remain active and take plenty of sensible exercise, not too strenuous, in clean fresh air in natural environments. Including walking, mild games of tennis, leisure snow skiing (mountain = yang), and so forth. Focusing on any pursuit that stimulates the lower limbs and torso as this will stimulate the relevant stomach and spleen/pancreas meridians. These energy channels run up and down through the legs to the feet, from and to the upper body.

Long baths, steam baths and saunas and any pursuit that causes too much sweating, are to be avoided because of the potential mineral loss in the perspiration.

Responsible sun bathing (sun = yang) and sea bathing (salt water = yang) will help. Avoiding artificial tanning as this done by a yin ultra violet light. If possible keeping away from swimming pools with treated water, due to the high chemical content, being yin and detrimental.

Tai Chi Chuan, Chi Kung, and to a lesser degree Yoga, if taught properly will build the internal energy, the chi, which in turn will improve and balance the endocrine system. Improving the yang hormone of insulin from the pancreas, as well as reinforcing the immune system which is produced by the yang internal energy. This yang chi is naturally engendered from midnight to midday. Therefore it is more productive to exercise early morning.

A simple but effective seated Chi Kung, besides being a general tonic, is to focus energy in the abdominal area. This reverse breathing exercise (*Refer to* Chi Kung 1 from Part 3), requires both hands to be placed together (P.8), with palms facing and covering the area just below the navel (CV.6). This will help rebalance the energy of the pancreas as well as naturally improving blood circulation. It will strengthen the cardio-vascular system, as well as stimulating the other viscera including the liver, kidneys and stomach which all play an essential, inter-related role in the homeostasis of the body. Thus helping the overall system to stabilise the diabetes. These exercises are most effective when the chi is circulating through the meridians associated with the spleen/pancreas and the stomach, between 7.00 am - 11.00 am. (GMT or local solar time). Preferably carried out in a quiet place where there is fresh clean air away from drafts. In spring and summer, the more yang seasons, this can be done outside, if possible facing the rising sun. Repeat as many times as convenient, perhaps spurred on by the pleasant side effects of this abdominal massage. Being a firming up of the tummy muscles besides aiding digestion and elimination of toxins.

Chi Kung that requires specific chi focusing is best carried out early morning for the above reasons and is helpful in improving the endocrine system. They should only be carried out when feeling well. This is detailed in Part 3 and the following Chi Kungs are beneficial for diabetics :- 1), 1a), 2), 3), 6), 7), 8) & 9). Vary the type to suit one's organism and attention span.

The abdomen can be massaged early morning by holding the 'anal tuck' (*See* Part 3) as if one is preventing the excretion of urine and faeces. Whilst squeezing and holding upwards, the muscles in that area, one massages the abdomen with the palms of joined hands (P.8.) in a clockwise then anticlockwise fashion in cycles of four.

Another method of stimulating the stomach and spleen energy channels is to firmly stroke up and down the legs first thing in the morning. Firstly stroke down the outer, firmer yang part of the legs, with the palms, in a single action. Then draw the hands back up along the inner, yin soft side of the legs. Repeat as many times as preferred. Besides invigorating the chi in the relevant meridians and internal organs, it will relieve any residual stiffness.

Always check with a medical practitioner if you are going to take herbal remedies whilst taking prescribed medicines.

Digestive Disorders – From Mouth Ulcers, Stomach Complaints To Bowel Trouble.

General Symptoms and Causes of Complaints of the Digestive System, with Suggested Remedial Action

The digestive system starts in the mouth and ends at the anus, being one continuous passage of miracles. Started when food and drink enter at the top, then separated and transformed at the centre, into life giving nutrients, with the waste products being eliminated at the bottom. This continuous connected view being the principle that forms the holistic, complementary approach to diagnosis and cure. In other words, what you put in, is what you get out. If the body does not discharge the waste products of digestion fully, toxins remain in the system. A simple, yet unfamiliar method of diagnosis to the average person, testifying as to the state of the body, is the colour and consistency of faeces and urine. Although this can be initially a bit off putting, it is a very useful health guide. If the faeces are hard and dark it indicates an overly yang diet which can cause a whole variety of constricting yang digestive complaints. Whereas if the faeces are loose and very light it shows the opposite a very yin condition. Ideally faeces should be firm having a brown sandy colour, with little odour. For example if one takes too much of the very yang herb of ginseng, the stools will become hard and dark, ending up very yang, regardless of food intake. An overly salty diet will do the same harm.

Food In, Diagnostic Colour Out

A similar context applies to the colour, texture and odour of urine, but much more variable because liquids are processed much faster by the body. If fluid intake is fairly normal between c.1-1½ of litres of liquid a day, with the urine being dark, the contents of the bladder are more yang, for a variety of reasons such as excess yang foods, or low liquid intake, toxin discharge after an illness or after a conscious detoxification including weight loss or change of diet. However if the urine is very clear it shows heavy liquid intake. If light, troubled and frequent, it could show high sugar levels or a yin condition of poor kidney function. Ideally urine should not smell acrid, sweet or acidic and should be a golden yellow colour in a healthy person.

An assorted mix of the colour spectrum and consistency will demonstrate the level of disharmonious food and liquid intake with the obvious results and the potential long term consequences on the body. If the colour and texture of urine and faeces are at the extremes for a week or more and persistent, remedial action must be taken. If unusual colour or blood appears in any discharge consistently one should approach a doctor for diagnostic tests. Have a urine test or take medical advice, but if these symptoms are present for a day or so, it is usually a sign of discharge after an illness, change of diet, environment or the body's natural ability to discharge toxins.

This means that all the disorders of the digestive system originate from the type and quantity of food and drink consumed, the way it is eaten and how it passes through the digestive system, aided and abetted by a disturbed psyche like stress. (*See* Stress Section).

Digestive Interface

The digestive tract is an interface, where the outer world meets the inner. Therefore poor intake will result in poor sustenance.

In Complementary Medicine, the face is a microcosmic image of the internal organs. The orifice of the mouth indicates the condition of the stomach and intestines. For example, cysts on the right side of the mouth indicate yin stomach trouble, being acidic, with the possibility of a stomach ulcer on the left side of the stomach. Whereas a cyst on the left side of the mouth shows a problem with the right side of the stomach.

Mouth

The upper lip is associated to the upper part of the digestive tract such as the oesophagus and in particular the stomach, whilst the bottom lip is linked to the intestines, thus the lips reflect the condition of these inner organs. If the lower lips are loose, the intestines will be loose, preventing healthy peristaltic action. Dry or chapped lips are a sign of poor digestion for a variety of reasons. Normally brought about by snatched convenience food, accompanied by too much of the wrong fluids (*Refer to* Yin Yang Diet). The colour of the lips show the overall condition of chi and blood quality. Ideally the lips should be a pinkish hue. When full red, it shows the body is under cardio-vascular pressure, caused by exercise or even after sexual activity, which if temporary are acceptable. Otherwise it is a warning of a circulatory disorder. (*Refer to* Heart Section).

The cosmetic trend to adorn the lips, usually carried out by women, is unconsciously born from this phenomenon. Bright red lips signalling potential sexual arousal and so forth. Whilst at the other end of the spectrum, a purplish colour is a sign of poor chi and blood flow, indicating a very yin condition which becomes extremely apparent before death occurs.

The tongue besides showing the condition of the heart (*See* Heart Section) reveals the plight of the stomach. When the tongue has an off white bloom or furred, the stomach is in trouble and food is not being digested properly. A clean pink tongue is a sign of good health. One must try to avoid eating late, preferably before 6.00 pm. (GMT or local solar time) because food is not easily or properly digested afterwards.

Time for Digestion

From midday to midnight the internal energy which is governed by solar time is waning, the nearer midnight the less effectual is the digestion. The later part of this circadian rhythm is not suitable for food assimilation because the internal energy is in its resting and healing phase.

It takes about three to six hours, depending on activity and the individual metabolic rate, for food to be passed along the 6.5 - 7.5 metres of the small intestine. This is where absorption of essential nutrients take place. Also peristalsis and digestion are more efficient in the yang chi phase before midday as opposed to the yin evening cycle.

The 'vibrational' energy pitch of food i.e. whether it is too yin or yang, also has a residual effect on the digestive tract because the energy of food can interfere with the nervous system.

Alcohol is yin, inducing dilation, being an anaesthetic on the nervous system. Hence the sloppy traits of a person who is under the influence of alcohol or drugs. All food and drink effect the nervous system in the same manner, albeit less evidently.

Chi and Digestion

The nervous system is fuelled by the electrical energy of the body, in turn controlling the peristaltic action of the gut. This is how the type and quality of food can drastically change the digestive function.

The parasympathetic nervous system, being yang, contracts the stomach and intestines whilst the sympathetic suppresses or yinnises peristalsis. This action squeezes the food along the digestive tract for effective digestion and elimination. Therefore if the food is too yin or yang besides its direct effect on the digestion, there is the resultant effect on the nervous system. This interferes with the assimilation and separation of the nutrients. Too much yin food will disturb the sympathetic nervous system and dilate the tract unnecessarily, whereas excess yang food will give rise to too much contraction, restricting the normal passage of nutrients.

All of the following are caused by excesses of yin and yang type foods and hectic lifestyle. This includes industrialised foods especially GMO's, which seem to disturb the digestive system, hence all the wheat allergies etc.. Mammoth producers of cereals such as the US, Canada, Russia, India and China have been growing GM crops for many years.

Cold Sores

Starting at the top of the digestive process, one of the most irritating oral complaints are cold sores. These are medically diagnosed as a herpes virus (HSV1). Cold sores are caused by erratic eating habits and or the transmission of the virus by contact with an infected third party, because the immune function is under par. A centred yin yang diet, including the immune boosting garlic, will fortify the immune system. Also creating the more acceptable, alkaline solution in the mouth. This helps reduce the frequency of the sores until such time as the immune function can deal with this yin virus. One can apply bicarbonate of soda, tinctures of Myrrh and Calendula or lemon juice, adjusting the frequency and type depending on effect, to the sore before retiring to relieve the symptoms. Echinacea will also boost the immune system, helping to eradicate the virus naturally. Rinsing the mouth and or brushing the teeth with a solution of sea salt will help ease the condition.

Mouth Ulcers

They are equally the fault of stress and or an unbalanced diet. An ulcerated mouth is in an acidic state instead of alkaline, caused by not chewing food properly. Aggravated by the over consumption of one or a mixture of the following acid generating substances from industrialised foodstuffs:- dairy produce, chocolate and sweets, sugar and sugar by products as in jam etc., soft drinks, citrus fruit drinks, too much fruit even if eaten in season, bananas, spices, tomatoes, pickles, potatoes, spinach, strong alcohol, regular tea and coffee, aspirin, drugs and so forth. All being yin 'acidic' elements.

Besides balancing diet away from yin acidic substances, the symptoms can be eased by rinsing one's mouth out with one teaspoon of 'pure' sea salt added to 25cls. of filtered warmed water. This can be carried out after eating and teeth brushing. Especially before retiring because this will leave a yang alkalising residue in the mouth. This will also yangise (close) the sore, assisting the natural healing process.(*See* Teeth Section).

Stomach & Peptic Ulcers

Both the gastric and the duodenal ulcers are the result of poor diet, insufficient chewing, intensified by stress. In Complementary Medicine the mouth and the stomach are linked to the emotion of anxiety, which is triggered by stress. The anxiety making the stomach produce an abundance of the yin gastric juice of hydrochloric acid (HCL), taking the stomach over the acid tolerance threshold.

Glands in the mucous-membrane lining of the stomach make and store an inactive protein called pepsinogen. The impulses from the vagus nerve (Jamen/GV.15 - *fig.14*) and the hormonal secretions of gastrin and secretin stimulate the release of pepsinogen into the stomach. Here it is mixed with hydrochloric acid and rapidly converted to the active enzyme pepsin. In a healthy person the gastric acids are neutralised in the intestine. The digestive power of pepsin is greatest at the acidity of normal gastric juice (pH 1.5-2.5). Poor diet will disrupt this process producing too much acidity thus producing a climate for ulcers.

Dry lips, sores in and around the mouth are a warning of stomach trouble ahead. This shows that the acidity of the stomach is rising to unmanageable levels for the body to cope with. Stomach ulceration occurs when the threshold of acid tolerance has been reached, rupturing the lining of the stomach. Giving rise to the symptoms of acute pain in the abdomen. Discomfort after a meal indicates a gastric ulcer, if the pain is acute before eating when the stomach is empty it verifies a duodenal ulcer.

If an ulcer is left to worsen without eliminating the cause, it can reach such a level that diet alone may not heal it. Drugs or surgery may be necessary to prevent the ulcer deteriorating further, thus preventing the symptoms of blood in the stools and haemorrhaging.

After this drastic action, although preventable if caught in time, a basic yin yang diet must be adhered to as this will fully heal any ulcer for the long term. However one must keep to a bias of well chewed grains and vegetables (*See* Yin Yang Diet). Taking care to avoid acidic foods including dairy foods, tropical and citrus fruit, sugar, spices, confection, coffee and alcohol, etc. i.e. the same taboo foods mentioned above in 'mouth ulcers'. The yin yang diet is more effective if the food is chewed into a pulp or blitzed into a soup. Barley water made from organic barley, boiled and sieved, then the liquid refrigerated for future use is helpful. Marshmallow root powder, aloe vera are also very effective at controlling the excess acid as well as aiding digestion, thus allowing the ulceration to heal. This will start the digestion in the mouth, thus lightening the load of the stomach. Then this dynamic vascular sac can function efficiently by mashing up and preparing the nutrients of food to be extracted and digested by the body correctly in the intestines. When the symptoms have passed and the ulceration has healed, one can cautiously experiment with foods, adjusting diet to suit taste and lifestyle. Liquorice, meadowsweet and aloe vera juice are soothing. Papaya fruit in small amounts, as well as the mastic gum derived from the pistachio tree will help heal the ruptures, also comfrey can be helpful in healing the damaged membranes. This can be assisted by a course of echinacea which will boost the immune function thus removing any harmful bacteria produced by the ulceration.

Selection of Disorders of the Intestines follows:-

Colitis

It is a painful inflammation of the large intestine giving rise to erratic bowel movements with diarrhoea (yin), and sometimes constipation (yang); often psychosomatic in origin. It is coupled by excess consumption of both yin and yang food i.e. (yang) poor quality animal protein hence constipation and more likely an excess of junk foods, spices and alcohol giving rise to loose yin bowel movement. A simple method to cure this is agar, agar being a seaweed that encourages peristalsis. Fresh greens and grains will put back useful bacteria in the bowel.

Irritable Bowel Syndrome (IBS)

This is diagnosed as encompassing the symptoms of heartburn, nausea, belching, abdominal pain, increased gas, irregular bowel movements including both diarrhoea and constipation, without the inflammation of colitis. The complaint of IBS is stimulated by excesses of yin and yang foods and or stress, giving rise to its episodic nature. This term has now become an umbrella for all mild yet irritating digestive disorders. A balanced, vegan yin yang diet will return the bowel to normal. Peppermint is one of the oldest and most successful herbs to clean the digestive system as well as reducing flatulence and aiding digestion. Occasional use of coriander and fennel in cooking as a mild seasoning will relieve the trapped wind caused by the symptoms of IBS and some foodstuffs. But remember these herbs are yin so must be used in minimal quantities as an aid to digestion, not as a cure because an unbalanced diet is the root cause.

Diverticulitis

This is a complaint when undigested food mixes with bacteria, both of which accumulate in a diverticulum or pouch in a weakened area of the gastrointestinal wall. The fetid food forms a hard mass called a fecalith. The fecalith reduces blood supply and infection occurs even giving rise to an abscess. Pain is usually felt in the lower left abdominal quadrant creating the symptoms of nausea, vomiting, low-grade fever and abdominal distention. This is basically a disorder that predominantly strikes the 'Western' male due to an over consumption of refined foods, poor quality animal protein, dairy produce, alcohol, spiced food and pollution. This cocktail induces the bowel to become lazy and flaccid reducing peristaltic action, causing the above symptoms. Because of the diversion in the bowel fasting one day a week would help clear and mend the diverticulum more quickly, coupled with reverse breathing (*See* Exercises and Massage Section) and a balanced yin yang diet. A diet of organic soups consisting of whole ground grains and vegetables with added garlic to ease bacteria will help return the bowel to its normal course. A course of echinacea will boost the immune system in order to remove any infection.

Crohn's Disease

This is characterised by diarrhoea, severe stomach pain, nausea, fever, chills, and weakness with weight and appetite loss being the general symptoms. The small intestine and or the main part of the colon are inflamed causing a thickening of the wall to the intestines, involved with extensive fibrosis and granulomas being patchy ulcerations that form on the mucosa. It is caused by a diet that lacks whole grain roughage and fresh seasonal vegetables triggered by either poverty or conversely overly rich foods. In 2003 Doctors cited that giving up smoking is a better cure than the drugs on offer. This is because the lung and large intestine energy or chi is linked, thus when the lung is functioning correctly its brother organ of the colon will heal more readily. High fibre consisting of organic grains especially brown rice allied with plenty of cooked greens, cutting out all sugar and sugar by products and junk food, will assist the colon to heal itself more rapidly. Thus the yin yang diet and sensible exercise clears up this complaint. (*See* Exercise and Massage Section).

Hernia

Normally diagnosed in males, the most common being a protrusion of an internal organ, usually the bowel, through an abnormal opening or weakness in the muscle wall. The causes include congenital malformation, traumatic injury, muscle weakening due to diet and or pregnancy, long-term heavy lifting, surgery, obesity, ascites (abnormal accumulation of abdominal fluid), abdominal tumour as well as aging. The latter, especially appertaining to an unbalanced diet that lacks roughage and or a diet of extremes of yin and yang, not only effect the nervous system, but weaken the salient muscle wall.

The general symptoms are a bulge in the inguinal (groin), femoral, or umbilical area or at an incision site if caused by surgery. The bulge may become larger with a shift in position or coughing, accompanied by a sharp, steady pain in the affected area. Signs of hernia strangulation include increasing severity of pain and fever, tachycardia, abdominal rigidity, and absence of bowel sounds. In severe cases surgery is needed. However a return to a yin yang diet will not only prevent any further trouble but also accelerate healing. Rubbing the abdomen as cited at the end of this section will strengthen the chi and the muscles of the whole abdomen. Especially after eating a balanced meal which has been well chewed, with limited liquid intake. Walking in fresh air fortifies the intestines thus helping to heal the hernia. (*See* Exercises and Massage Section).

Colon and Rectal Cancer

These are still prevalent today despite the fact that doctors realised years ago that a diet of refined foods is one of the main causes. In 1969 I was watching my black and white television in my student digs when an eminent Harley Street surgeon and consultant appeared on the BBC News warning the viewers that most colon and rectal cancer was caused by a diet of refined foods. He cited the 'white wonder loaf' and a lack of roughage as the main cause. This triggered me into a whole new way of looking at food, besides instigating from that day on, the buying of organic whole grain bread. This occurred as I was exposed to the yin yang principles of diet and exercise.

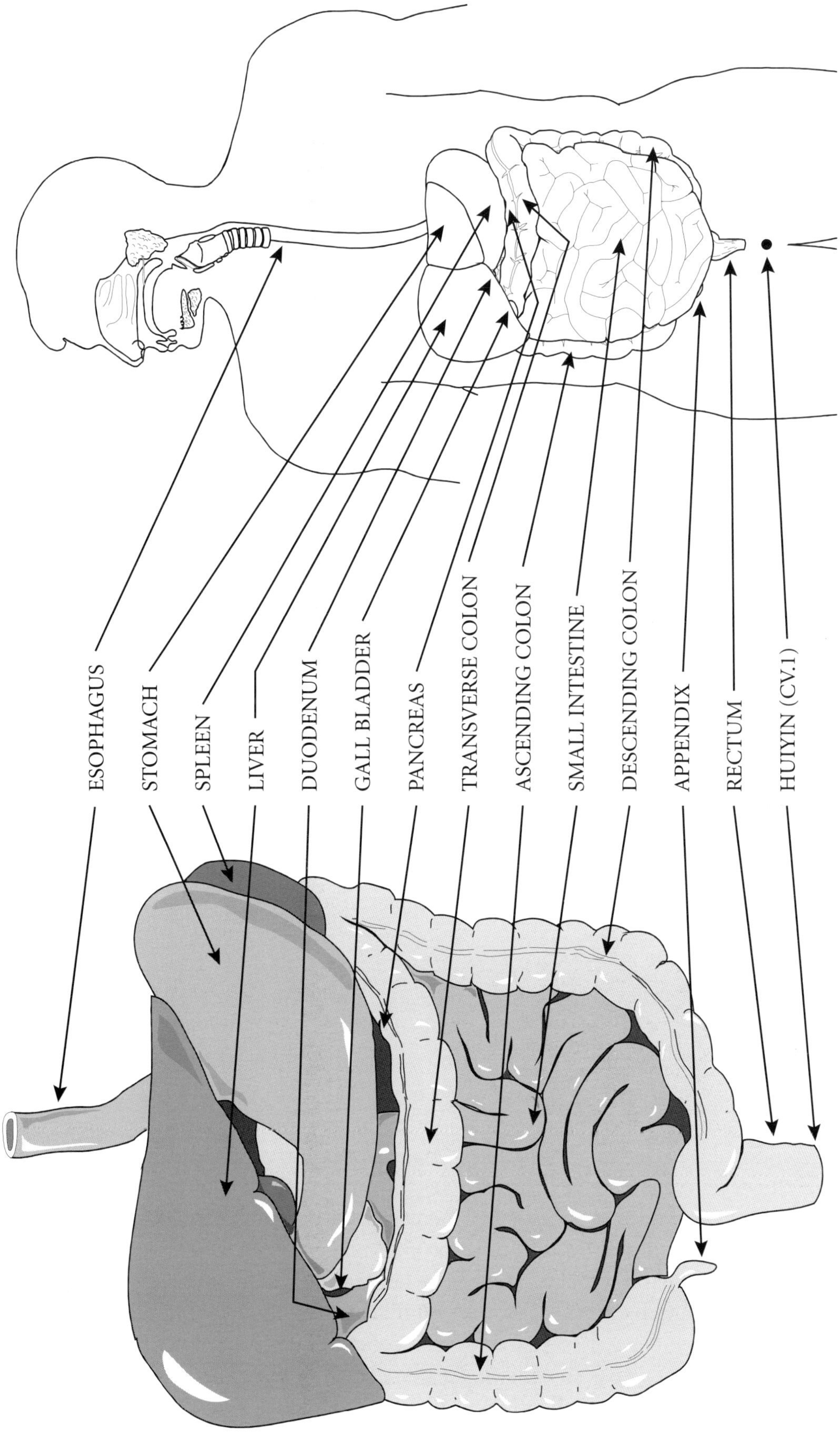

Figure 4: **Digestive Tract.**

Life has become much more complicated since that time with the increase of factory farming, pollution, smoking (in Complementary Medicine the intestines are connected to the lungs and the heart, therefore if these organs are weakened there is a quid pro quo effect on the digestive tract.), prescribed drugs, stress, misuse of antibiotics and so forth. If the cancer is diagnosed early enough a program of self-awareness, a yin yang diet, internal energy exercises such as Tai Chi, Chi Kung and Yoga can possibly clear the cancer. These balancing methods will also heal the after effects of a cancer acting as a future safeguard as well. It would have to be in co-operation with a sympathetic medical structure such as to be found at the Bristol Clinic, Devon England. This clinic adopts an holistic approach, taking into consideration, diet, stress, lifestyle, allied to chi balancing exercises such as Tai Chi Chuan, Chi Kung and Yoga which would assist the return of the healing energy to the affected tissues.

Cancer and Fate

Dr. Carl Jung realised in the 1940's that cancer could be a form of mental repression as well. The cancer, being the negative result of a repressed content, manifesting itself in the body. In other words a disturbed psyche. Nowadays there is a new collective threat of cancer which is allied to pollution, nuclear fall out, pesticides, chemical additives in food and drink and so forth. These being a form of collective neurosis, where mankind is playing at being God, thus having collective clusters and results. Unfortunately a combination of the two, can be fatal.

This is the reason, as in all diseases, that a holistic approach is needed to cure any illness. Therefore a formula of balancing food, the psyche and lifestyle is needed. There are chi exercises that help heal the area as well.

For example to energise increase to the flow of blood and healing energy to the rectum, holding the anal tuck is a very useful method of assisting healing in this area. (*See* Exercise and Massage Section). The anal tuck can be repeated all day and whenever you can. It will also stimulate and prevent stagnation of the chi in the prostrate in men and the cervix in women. This is very beneficent for rectal cancer whilst practicing the following Chi Kungs from Part 3 - 1), 1a), 6), 7) & 8).

Yin and Yang and Cancer

To illustrate how yin yang is related to cancer of the colon; cancer of the ascending colon, being a relatively more yin part of the intestine is generally caused by a poor quality yin diet. Whereas the transverse and descending colons are relatively more yang, the cancer here probably engendered by relatively more yang 'chaotic' foods. The rectum being the most yang area of the digestive system is disturbed by yang food which will create this area to become unusually yang and restricted. So if there is a cancer tendency, an abundance of unbalanced yang industrialised foods such as animal protein, in particular red meat and fast food derivatives, such as burgers particularly when barbecued or smoked, over yangises food. Also dairy food, salty foods and so forth will increase the tendency to cause cancer of the rectum (*See* Yin Yang Diet). Residual toxins including pesticides, insecticides, artificial fertilisers in fruit and vegetables also aid and abet cancer, as do GMO's.

Therefore a strict organic vegan diet based on the yin yang diet, which can be fine tuned by eating more acceptable yin food for the yang cancers and more yang for the yin. Initially the yin yang diet can be blended into soups with an emphasis on greens, seaweed and garlic to rest and clear the gut.

For example if we take the average principle of 70% yang of grains to 30% yin of vegetables and liquid. Therefore if there is a yang cancer of the rectum, one should moderate the yang grains down to 50% and so forth, always keeping pure fluid intake to a minimum. But there is no risk if one adjusts 15-20% either way because the yin yang diet is very safe and balanced anyway. It can never harm, only heal. So the degree of yin yang adjustment is just another way of improving the restorative process.

An absolute essential is to try and abstain from the all industrialised yin yang extremes in diet, because they are a material catalyst for the cancer. Remember Jung's maxim that 'the body is the mere visibility of the soul and the soul is the psychological experience of the body'. Therefore despite any healing system, complementary or standard, deep reflection is needed and a quid pro quo with the unconscious for the disease to be remedied with the answer being found in the troubled soul. (*See* Stress Section and ***Time for a Change***).

Haemorrhoids

Or piles are an enlarged vein in the lower rectum or anus caused by blockage in the veins of this area. Internal haemorrhoids begin above the internal opening of the anus. If they become large enough to protrude from the anus, they become squeezed and painful. Small internal haemorrhoids may bleed with bowel movements. External haemorrhoids appear outside the anal opening. They are usually not painful, and bleeding does not occur unless a haemorrhoidal vein breaks or becomes blocked.

Haemorrhoids are aggravated by over straining when defecating, constipation and too much sitting will also encourage them. Pregnancy can help bring on haemorrhoids, so pregnant women are advised to eat plenty of roughage in a balanced diet.

Western Medical treatment includes the use of surface medication to lubricate, kill the pain, and shrink the haemorrhoid. The haemorrhoids may need to be hardened by injection, tied off, or removed by a surgical procedure, including laser treatment; tying off is becoming the more preferred medical treatment. It is simple, effective, and does not require anaesthesia. The haemorrhoid is grasped with forceps and a rubber band is slipped over the enlarged part, causing the tissue to die and the haemorrhoid to fall off, usually within a week.

Haemorrhoids are caused by an excess consumption of yin or yang foods. Therefore a diet which is too yin will cause the capillaries of the blood vessels in the rectum to expand and rupture. Therefore avoid the yin dilating foods of fruit, salads, cold liquids, especially soft drinks, tea, coffee, ice cream, confection and sugar products, raw vegetables, spices, acidic foods like vinegar and citrus fruits. Whereas an over consumption of yang foods such as red meat, dairy food, eggs and fish, salt and salt by products such as TV snacks, crisps etc., will make the blood vessels contract too much. Thus causing the unpleasant and alarming symptoms of bleeding. Haemorrhoids are caused by the above factors because of a weakness in that area due to a poor diet or lifestyle maintained over a long time. To cure haemorrhoids completely, one must eat a centred yin yang diet ensuring to chew food properly, keeping away from extremes until the piles are healed.

Herbs

Herbs and Plants etc. that are helpful for haemorrhoids include rutin in tablet form, comfrey and chestnuts used as a food supplement, 'real' natural liquorice (check ingredients on labels because proper liquorice is usually only found in health food shops). Soothing 'external' application can be applied to the affected area using Witch Hazel or Pilewort which are both calming as well as helping to reduce the haemorrhoids. These remedies can also be used in hip baths and cold or hot packs which are also soothing, when applied around the area of the piles.

The following Chi Kungs from Part 3 will help the healing energy and correct blood flow to the affected area of the piles. Being 1), 1a), 2), 6), 7), 8) & 9), these should be carried out, whilst holding the anal tuck, (*See* Exercise and Massage Section). The anal tuck exercise can be repeated on its own, all day or whenever convenient, this will encourage healing chi and blood to the rectum.

General Exercise and Massage for the Entire Digestive System

A variety of Chi Kungs are excellent for the whole digestive system being 1), 1a), 2), 3), 6), 7), 8) & 9) which will have more benefit if practised in the morning.

The two main meridians that feed chi to the relevant nervous systems, are the Water channel of the Dumo and the Fire channel of Renmo (*fig.14*). The chi of these channels feeds the nervous and digestive systems. There are several Chi Kungs in this book which will help the chi to stimulate the various parts of the nervous system. Including the vagus nerve at the Jamen, (GV.15) on the base of the hairline on the back of the neck as well as the sympathetic nervous complex around the solar plexus (CV.6 - *fig.14*). The recommended Chi Kungs to stimulate these and other channels are:- 1), 1a), 2), 3), 7) & 8), from Part 3.

Rest and Digestion

Always allow thirty to sixty minute gap between eating or drinking and Chi Kung. Reverse breathing 1) & 1a) are the exception as these can be practised all the time to help heal the complaint or when discomfort is felt, as it will massage and stimulate the salient organs and their chi.

Fasting once a week is very helpful in aiding to clear up digestive complaints, allowing the system to rest and heal.

Anal Tuck

The 'anal tuck' is a physical and chi stimulus to strengthen the lower gut as well as acting as a plug and energiser of this lower chi gate, called the Huiyin (CV.1 - *fig.14*). This acupoint is used to circulate chi up the spine as well as preventing a leakage of energy by way of the anal sphincter, thus holding chi in this area.

To perform the anal tuck one gently holds the muscles of the rectum taught, in and upwards, as if one is preventing oneself from going to the toilet, for a minute or so, or preferably as long as one can. Then release them. The hold and release of the anal tuck can also be done in gentle rapid bursts, about one full contraction and a release, each second.

Another beneficial exercise is to hold the anal tuck, whilst massaging the abdomen with the exposed palm of hands resting on each other, with the centre of the palms aligned. (P.8. - *fig.21*). The palm of the hand massages the tummy in a clockwise then anticlockwise fashion.

Early Tai Chi, Yoga, and Exercise

Chi Kung, Tai Chi and Yoga are excellent for balancing the internal energy of the organism. Also one should take regular exercise that is not too strenuous like walking, leisure cycling, swimming, tennis and so forth. All of which will help keep the digestive system in good repair.

Conclusion

If one experiences trouble in the body, the cause is to found in the food, environment, lifestyle and stress. All of which have to be considered together to effect a cure.

It is more beneficent to perform any exercise including Chi Kung and Tai Chi in the morning. This is because the circadian status of chi in the morning is yang which builds and protects, it is also the time that chi energises the intestines and the stomach, before midday. Never rush or gulp meals, be continental and take your time, enjoy the food. Whenever possible eat with friends or family. However, always in a convivial way in a pleasant environment. Following the old saying, 'Breakfast like a king, lunch like a prince and dine like a pauper' being timeless wisdom. Eat what you drink and drink what you eat is a wise old Chinese proverb, i.e. chew food well and do not drink too much fluid.

The digestive system responds immediately to the quality of food input, with all the various symptoms laid out above which can only worsen if not reversed. All being relative warning signs of an unbalanced diet and lifestyle.

Stress as well as interfering with one's general demeanour will give rise to the residual anxiety having an immediate yang tightening effect on the digestive system and the circulation, thus restricting nourishment.

A balanced yin yang diet will remedy the energy input differentials, being a tried and tested way of centring this process, coupled with a balanced lifestyle will help to restore the overall homeostasis and health of the mind and body.

Initially one should ensure to eat more before midday. The diet should be a grain vegan diet as laid out in the yin yang diet. As stated brown rice contains phytin acid which is excellent at removing toxins naturally from the body especially the stomach and bowels. Also turning the food into a gruel or soup, keeping the same proportions as in the yin yang diet will speed up recovery of all digestive disorders, regardless of gravity.

Always check with a medical practitioner if you are going to take herbal remedies whilst taking prescribed medicines.

Eye Complaints and Syndromes with Remedial Exercises

Science and Soul

The purely anatomical view of the eye shows this intricate structure to be a sense organ which transforms light images into electrical charges that the brain translates into the picture format, which sighted people take for granted. This singular view creates a caveat for modern science as it does not formally recognise the internal energy, chi, of the human being. Yet everybody is aware that the eye has more functions than just perceiving objects in a one directional manner, i.e. inwards only.

The eyes emanate emotional criteria displaying moods of sadness, joy, anxiety, fear, anger and so forth. This phenomenon is also clearly apparent in animals. This factor is confirmed by references in literature and traditions from all cultures in every period of history. Our forbears were aware that a look or regard contained an expression of inner feelings. The evil eye or a glad eye has nothing to do with the mechanics of vision itself. Whereas body language can be controlled to cover up emotions, the eye cannot lie, hence the expression 'look me in the eye when you say that'.

Skilled interrogators from the secret services and the police are trained to catch the response from the eye when questioning suspects. This accepted subtle ability is the way in which one can actually espy the intimate energy of another with one's own internal sensors. The ancient Chinese Masters were there before us, adopting the Taoist doctrine of opposites, they reasoned that if there were five outer senses then there must be five inner ones. They are linked and motivated by the internal energy of the mind and body, which they called inner breath or chi (*See* Part 3 for a description of chi).

Inner Senses

Even at the beginning of the twenty first century neurologists are also studying this mysterious phenomenon. They have discovered a 'blindsight'. This paradoxical term describes the phenomenon when a registered blind person can 'see' objects held in front of him or her. This fact that the blind can 'see', cannot be explained by orthodox science. If we return to the Taoist logic of a double edged sense, it becomes conceivable that there is an inner sight capable of visualising outer objects as well. The scientists conducting this study at a leading London teaching hospital discovered that when they drew the attention of blind volunteers to this blindsight, some of them became confused and disturbed because they 'saw' things.

This peculiar phenomenon also applies to the other senses which are now labelled as unconscious senses. They appear to act as a back up to the five outer ones. A similar effect happens to individuals who have lost their sense of touch due to nerve damage, with a 'numb touch'. The senseless limbs can feel a pin prick or heat even under clinical conditions. Also the clinically deaf can mysteriously identify sounds with their 'deaf hearing'. Maybe this is how Beethoven could compose his extraordinary music even after he became stone deaf. The inner sense of smell can also be utilised. After a road accident where I suffered extensive facial damage, my olfactory nerve was completely damaged. The plastic surgeon said that I would lose my sense of smell. Although I seemed to have lost my regular sense of smell,

Irises pointing in abnormally, indicate a sign of being too yang with potential high blood pressure and acidosis.

Irises that face out indicate an overly yin condition with blood being too alkaline and a tendancy towards yin cancers.

One iris pointing in, whilst one is normally centred can indicate diabetes.

Low set irises indicate a very yang condition, noticeable and normal in babies but in adults can indicate cruelly and even madness.

High set irises are a very yin condition seen in the infirm, people with poor reflexes and or the elderly.

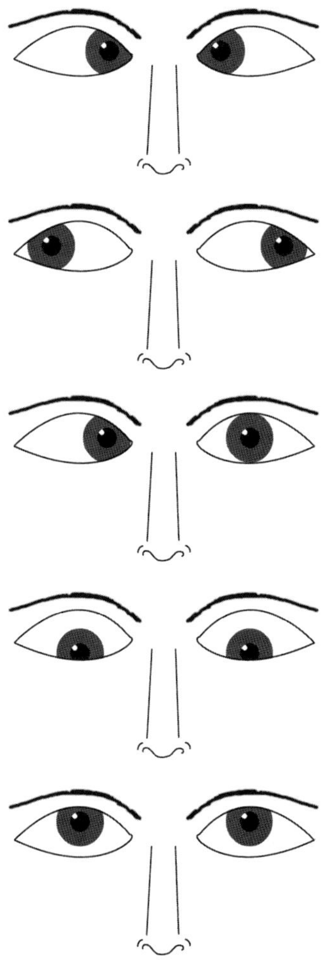

Figure 5: It is the internal energy or chi that gives rise to the various effects in the body, clearly perceptible in the positioning of the eyes, yin having an outward or upward and dilatory effect, whereas yang causes an inward or downward result and contraction.

often without any particular focus I have 'ghost' smells where I can sense coffee, perfume, tobacco or petrol etc.. However if I concentrate I can smell things, albeit less intensely than I used to.

Ghost Limbs

Another proof of these inner senses happened to me whilst I was recovering in hospital at the plastic surgery unit of the Queen Victoria Hospital in East Grinstead, Sussex. A fellow patient, a charming cockney despite having lost one leg, used to ask me to scratch his 'left leg', which had been amputated. He assured me that he felt sensations in the area of his invisible limb which would itch from time to time. When the expected place of the illusory limb was rubbed, it would relieve the irritation. Presumptuously I asked an experienced nurse to explain why this chirpy, yet unfortunate lad had these bizarre sensations. My impudent question was just shrugged off, by informing me that it happened a lot to these 'ghost limbs'.

It took another ten years to discover the reason for this, when I became enlightened by studying acupuncture which showed how 'chi', the body's internal energy, runs bilaterally down both legs. The energy will continue to circulate down these ghost limbs even though a physical limb could be missing. The chi was still flowing along both the invisible channels of my one legged friend.

The spirit of this inner sight is the mind's eye. This inner sense organ is used to muse over past visual experiences of places, people and so forth. This 'third eye' was considered by the influential seventeenth century mathematician and philosopher, Réné Descartes, to be housed in the pineal gland. He is most renowned for *"Cogito ergo sum"* - *"I think therefore I am"*. This inner eye can 'see' dreams and visions, which are usually the first encounter with the inward world of the unconscious as well as being an essential medium for the true journey of the soul.

This phenomenon was studied and explained in depth by Professor Carl Jung, which he laid out in his collected works. Dr. Jung superseded the more superficial Freudian approach to this secret world of truth which discarded its depth in an intellectual manner, leaving Jung to delve and interpret its unique message. The unconscious can also communicate its message by the other inner senses of hearing, smell, touch and taste. One only has to reflect the impact a dream can impart by way of these inner senses which can be as dramatically engaged, and in some cases more so than, the effects of any outer experience.

Inspiration, Soul and Spirit

This internal energy is the actual motivation for life itself and it is not by chance that there is a saying that the eye is the window of the soul. The advances in medical procedures on the mechanics of the eye are improving all the time but all medical cures rely on the natural ability of the body to heal itself which is accomplished by this inner 'breath' or chi. Chi has parallels in many languages, one being soul, derived from the German 'seele' which is akin to 'gheist' both meaning spirit, Lt. 'spiritus' (in'spire' etc.) or breath. Hence the figurative or actual implication of the eye being a window to the inner breath of the soul. Again there are sayings such as; 'he has given up the ghost' implying that the grip on life has been lost, giving the person a vacant look in his or her eyes.

In Complementary Medicine the eye is linked to the energy of the Liver and Gall Bladder which the Chinese Alchemists considered to be the night time residence of the soul, even the English word 'liver' is derived from the word 'live' because their Western counterparts also believed that the spirit dwelt there.

Whether the alchemists of either culture were right or wrong is a consideration left to the imagination of the individual. However an empirical truth from the same oriental discipline shows a medically sound diagnosis to assess the condition of liver energy. The ability of the eyes to cope with bright light at night or early morning is determined by the strength of the liver chi. If weak or yin, the eyes will be more yin and effected by the relative yang strength of the light and so forth. After a late night accompanied by alcohol, both of which deplete liver chi, the eyes are much more sensitive, because the liver has been yinnised by a lack of rest coupled by the onslaught of a yin substance like alcohol. Liver chi is replenished during its period of recharge occurring between 11. p.m. and 3.00 a.m. (GMT or local solar time). This is when the daily cycle of chi runs through the meridians of the liver and gall bladder respectively. Therefore if one is active or the liver is under pressure at this time, the chi will not be able to accomplish its circadian function of re-balancing the energy of these organs. This in turn will effect vision because the meridians of the gall bladder and the liver are two of the main channels which are responsible for the energy of the eyes. When the chi of the mind and body is depleted (*See* Part 3) this will effect the energy level of the eye making it more difficult to focus clearly. General eyesight is also conditioned by liver chi.

The position of the eyes can indicate the condition of the internal energy. When the eyes are set high in their sockets, it is because the eyeball is expanded, being a sign of an extreme yin physiology. When a white crescent is clearly visible under the eyes, people in this extreme condition are more prone to accidents and danger. Whereas a low set eyeball is due to a smaller shape, this condition is normal for babies, but during ensuing growth, the eyes of the infant should naturally centre themselves into the normal position. If a mature individual has white clearly visible above the eyes, it is a sign of an overly yang constitution, causing the individual to display irrational anger and violence. It is clearly visible in the disturbed or insane. Both conditions are due to excess exposure of extremes of yin and yang substances in diet, drugs, or the environment and emotional disturbance. (*fig.5*).

Last but not least is the pupil which can be permanently dilated whilst taking drugs or during a trauma. Besides the chemical yinnisation, it is a sign of the organism wanting more light or awareness, hence the opening of the iris. Any form of repression, whether a self induced banishment of a problem held down by will power or chemically motivated, cannot heal permanently. The only long term cure is to face the problem, however awful it may appear because the answer lies at the heart of the problem. Albeit at one's own pace. An honest open heart will allow the healing aspect of the unconscious to permeate into the conscious field. Thus ensuring a complete cure.

Iridology

This is a study of the eye which basically considers, that the eye is a microcosmic mirror of the body, in a similar way that the feet in reflexology reflect the organism. Generally speaking the upper parts of the white of the eye relate to the upper parts of an individual and so forth. Any discoloration or marks indicate problems in the related areas of the person. A quick colour guide of the white of the eye shows general organ problems which is as follows: a yellowing of the white of the eye indicates liver and gall bladder malfunction, a dark hue shows that the kidneys have been under long term pressure whereas a reddening can alert one to heart and circulation problems.

Eyestrain and Computers

This new type of eyestrain is triggered by two interconnecting factors. Firstly the eye has to keep a rigid focus at the same distance for extended periods, coupled by the emissions from the screen which can damage the retina. Flat screens reduce the potential harm whereas VDU's are cathode ray tubes which fire electrons at the screen with harmful residual effects on the retina. One can relieve the eye strain of rigid focusing in situ whilst at one's computer as follows :- Initially try not to work continually for long periods at the screen, preferably no more than an ½ hour at a time without a break for the eye: from time to time exercise the eye with a purposeful change of focus by fixing one's vision on objects that are at a distance,

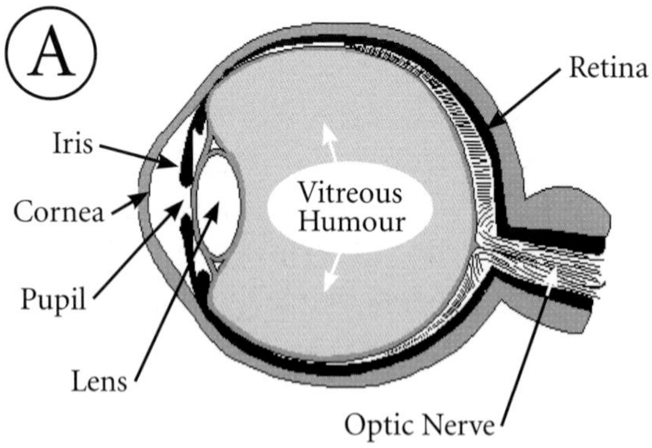

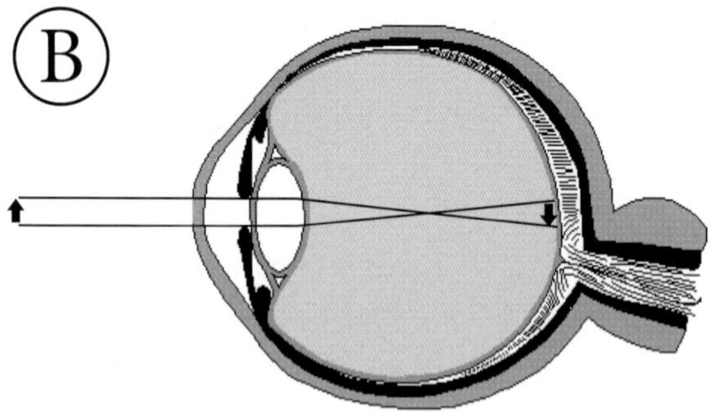

When the body is balanced, the vision will be normal with the image focusing directly onto the retina.

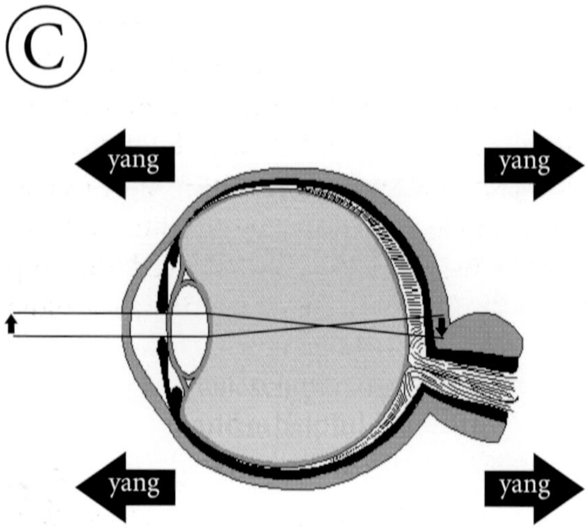

When the body energy is more yang, it can make the eyes more spherical or smaller, hence the image overshoots the retina, causing long sightedness.

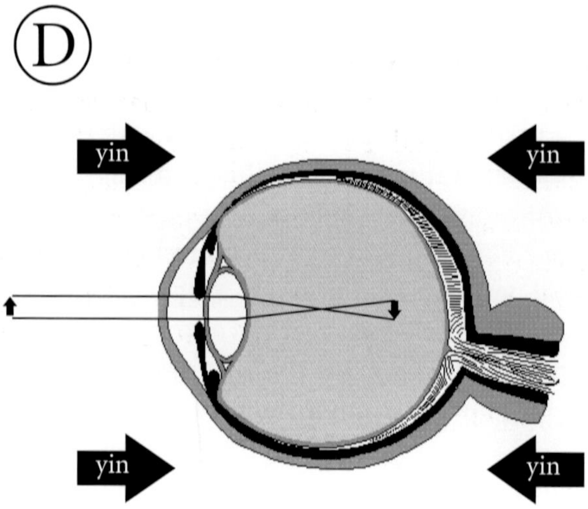

When the body energy is more yin, it can cause the lens of the eye to flatten, making the image fall short of the retina, causing short sightedness.

Figure 6: Excesses of yin/yang cause the eyes to distort e.g. diet, stress, VDU's, drugs, alcohol etc.. However an overall expanded eyeball, a yin energy condition, will also make the image fall short of the retina as in D, causing myopia. Whereas an overall contracted eyeball, being an excess yang energy condition, will give rise to hyperopia as in C, where the image overshoots the retina.
The main set of vital organs and their related internal energy to control the shape of the lens and the eye are the liver and gallbladder. (*See* Detox and Eye Sections).

then straight away to something nearby. This will also help the myopia which can be caused by extensive near screen or same distance focusing.

Always ensure that you have a reputable make of eye guard over the VDU screen which will help reduce the impulses from the cathode-ray tube of the monitor. Also try and do the eye exercises from this section, regularly.

Shortsightedness - Myopia

This is where the light from an object entering the eye falls short of the retina, caused by a reshaping of the eye or lens, thus changing the focal distance (*fig.6*). This usually occurs because the chi that controls the eye has become more yin causing a horizontal effect. If the eyes are in fairly good condition without any permanent damage this can be rectified by centring the chi which in turn will balance eye energy. This can be achieved by adhering to the yin yang diet and performing the eye exercises regularly. (*See* Eye Exercises *fig.7*).

Longsightedness - Hypermetropia

This describes the visual condition when light from an object overshoots the retina because the eyeball is yangised, smaller than necessary for normal focusing. (*fig.6*). Babies and the old have this condition naturally. Firstly babies are by nature more yang and compact after birth. Whereas the chi in the old has waned giving rise to the diminishing consequence of energy loss and thus long sightedness. If hypermetropia happens in between these stages, it is usually because the person is too yang. This gives rise to a shrinking of the eyeball due to over consumption of too much yang food especially, salty foods, animal protein and so forth (see Yin Yang Diet). Long sightedness can be greatly ameliorated with a balanced yin yang diet and eye exercises. Both of which will regulate the chi flow to the nerves and in turn allow the shape of the eye to resolve itself. (*See* Eye Exercises *fig.7*).

Colour Blindness

This is usually caused by extremes of yin and yang in the diet. If the red or orange yang spectrum is unclear or not discernible, it is due to too many yang substances being ingested. Whereas if blue or green colours are not visible, the diet is excessively yin with over indulgence of sugar, alcohol, spices and chemical additives etc.. If no permanent damage has occurred to the visual process, balancing food intake vis á vis the yin yang diet with determination using the eye exercises explained below, can clear the problem completely. Colour blindness can also be linked to a trauma. For example I knew a superficially pleasant man who worked in insurance who was colour blind, yet later ran off and left his family.

Sunglasses

Lenses of the right type, are a useful protection when worn appropriately. However if they are worn indiscriminately they can make the eyes lazy, actually weakening vision. Sunglasses should only be worn if the eyes are exposed to bright light, particularly the very yin 'blue light'. This is usually encountered in the rarer atmospheres of high altitudes or the poles, with the added danger of light refraction from the snow. This dangerous type of refraction also occurs at sea and over sand where these rays of the 'blue light' spectrum are prevalent. Blue light which can damage the lens, the cornea and the retina of the eye, can also occur whilst driving particularly, in sunny countries.

However the price of a pair of sunglasses does not guarantee correct filtration of harmful rays. One must research the type and quality of the sunglasses, determining their level of filtration which should be clearly indicated and guaranteed. The potentially damaging ultraviolet light can extend from 290-400 nanometers in fairly average conditions with the more extreme environment of blue light ranging from 400-510 nanometers. If a person has a yin diet or is in a yin condition from taking antibiotics for example, the eyes will be more yin and thus more prone to damage.

The lighter the colour of the eye, the more yin, the less defence it has against strong light. Hence blue eyed people have tended to evolve in the Northern climates where light levels are generally less, prior to ozone layer depletion. This process of natural evolution also developed the eye to become relatively darker nearer the equator. This natural yang mechanism of self-defence was engendered as protection from the more prolonged exposure to the harsher rays of the sun, giving rise to the dark brown eye of the tropics. Whereas the lighter brown eye has evolved to cope with a four season climate as has the variety of eye colours.

Crossed Eyes

If pointing inward, are a sign of excess yang intake or yang closed attitude. However if the eyes turn out then the opposite is the case, the person being too yin. If one eye turns in and one out then it indicates excesses of yin and yang. This condition is often prevalent in heavy drinkers (yin) who eat a lot of meat (yang). It can also be caused by an overload of sugary (yin) and salty (yang) foodstuffs. The remedy for all three is to centre the food in accordance with the procedures of the yin yang diet, accompanied by eye exercises at the end of this section. This condition can also be caused by stress and or diet. The eye exercises cited below and centring of diet can cure this syndrome.

Stye

This condition is a small boil of the sebaceous gland on the lid of the eye. This is caused when the blood has become stagnant due to consumption of excesses of either yin or yang type food and an infection has not been fought off. If the immune system is under par, the eyelid can be infected by a variety of microbes to be found in everyday life. Women should also be careful as some eye makeup has preservatives added to the cosmetic which can also irritate the eyes. Equally a cross infection can occur by applying old eye makeup. To cure a stye one has to strengthen the immune system by adhering to the yin yang diet, slightly increasing garlic which boosts the immune system helping clear up the blood. Avoiding all excesses especially alcohol, spices, sugar and dairy food. Two herbal preparations that help clear up eye infections are echinacea and eyebright which are available in herbalists and health food stores. To ease the external symptoms of eye irritation, applications of aloe vera juice or gel, and elderflower water will both help heal the complaint. To soothe the area one can also apply a cooled camomile tea bag over the eye.

Cataracts

They appear as a blue grey film usually over the crystalline lens or its capsule, blurring vision and can end with blindness. Cataracts often accompany diabetes, glaucoma, uraemia and kidney failure. They take a long time to develop and are generally caused by a diet of over expansive yin foods such as sugar, coffee, citrus fruit, potent drugs (steroids), alcohol, dairy food, spices and so forth. Also they can form if the diet is rich in saturated fats from dairy food and animal protein. Cataracts, as well, can form due to continued exposure to UV or blue light catalysed by the aforementioned reasons. In the southern hemisphere of South America which also suffers ozone layer depletion, a lot of sheep in Patagonia are blind with cataracts due to their exposure to the unfiltered UV light.

Cataracts can be reversed if one adheres to the balanced yin yang diet, especially avoiding the saturated fats of animal protein and the yin expansive foods mentioned earlier.

An age-old cure for cataracts is to add two teaspoonfuls of organic cider vinegar in a glass of warm filtered water, drunk twice a day before meals. Being careful not to overdue the cider vinegar because it is yin, and too much would be counter productive as well as weakening the organism.

A couple of drops of organic filtered sesame oil (heat sesame oil gently and filter through fine muslin, allow to completely cool), administered by a dropper to the eyes before retiring, will help reduce the cataract. Another natural external aid, is to take five to ten drops of fresh juice of the plant Greater Celandine to four tsp. of the distilled extract of witch hazel, diluted by one tsp. of a warm solution of pure filtered water. Put in an eye bath to douche the eyes three time a day, before eating. The eye exercises from this section will increase chi and blood flow to the area also helping to heal the cataract.

Conjunctivitis

This is an inflammation of the mucous membrane of the eye, the conjunctiva, can be caused by bacteria or allergens as in hay fever, or environmental irritants such as dust, smoke, noxious gases etc.. Symptoms include red eyes with intense itching, swelling of the lid, clear discharge, tearing, light sensitivity and sometimes a feeling of burning.

If conjunctivitis is triggered by an infection, firstly one has to clean up the blood as per the yin yang diet trying to avoid animal foods, dairy products and yin foodstuffs like sugar, chocolate, alcohol, excess liquid, coffee, spices which all reduce the immune function. Garlic boosts the immune system naturally, but as garlic is yin, over consumption will reverse its beneficial properties. Echinacea, a magic plant discovered by Cherokee and Mohawk North American Indians observed it would remove toxins from the body such as snake's venom. Studies have shown it to increase white blood cells, activating T-cells, stimulating the 'killer' cells that protect the organism from foreign bacteria. All of which improve the immune function considerably, being another useful way to help clear up infections. To ease the irritating symptoms apply externally or as an eye bath: four parts extract of distilled witch hazel diluted by one part warm pure filtered water. Also external applications of pure or organic aloe vera juice or gel to the lid are soothing and healing. Another suggestion is one tsp. of elderflower, or eyebright or camomile, infused in a mug of pure filtered boiled water (1/2 pint). Then allow the mixture to infuse for c. fifteen minutes which can be used in an eye bath. A fresh bath for each eye; a warm camomile teabag over the effected eye is a readily available and soothing application.

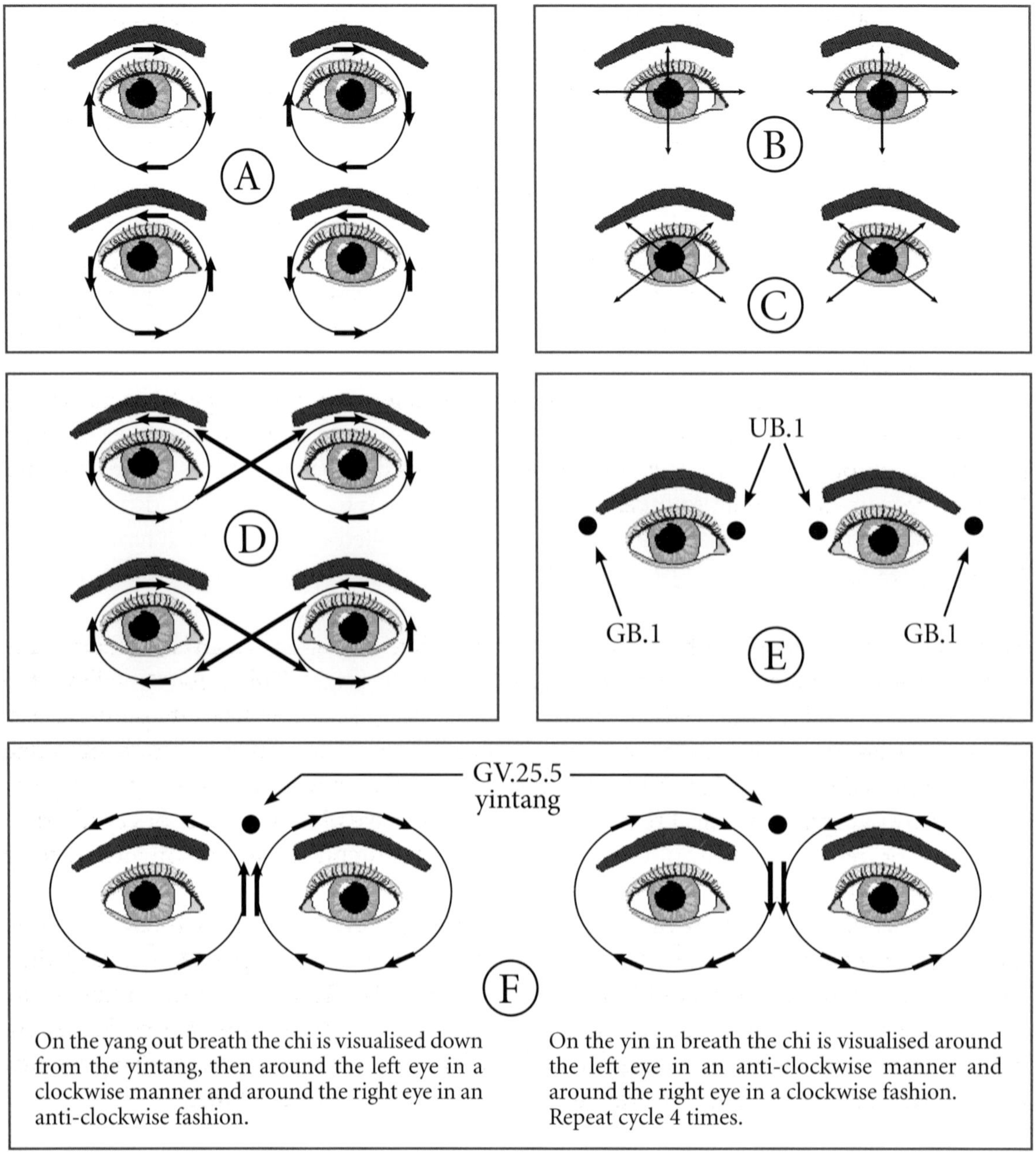

Figure 7

Glaucoma

This is a swelling and high pressure of the eyeball because of the imbalance of the inflow and outflow of the aqueous humour. The imbalance of this fluid that flows in through the pupil and out through the meshwork at the juncture of the iris and cornea, is caused by absorption of overly yin expansive substances in the form of sugar, strong drugs, alcohol, spices, citrus fruits, dairy foods and of course too much liquid. If left untreated glaucoma leads to progressively diminishing vision, degeneration of the optic nerve, and even blindness.

Surgery is often used to drain off some of the aqueous humour but as the cause is not addressed it will return. Therefore one has to centre the constitution because this is also a sign of severe yinisation of the organism. Firstly one must centre the energy of the body with the yin yang diet to prevent over production and retention of the aqueous humour. The natural healing process will be greatly assisted with the aid of natural diuretics like dandelion, nettle, burdock and fennel, ensuring to limit all liquid intake to ½ - ¾ of a litre a day until the pressure is removed from the eyeball.

This will become evident by medical measurements also by the improvement of the visual function, and the loss of the feeling of tightness of the eye. Careful doses of ginseng will help yangise the sufferer and help reduce the fluid trapped in the eye. But as glaucoma often happens in old people, the amount of ginseng has to be monitored. Because the elderly are naturally more contracted and ginseng can encourage a general overall tightness of limbs and muscles, if too much is taken.

French herbalists recommend an eye wash of diluted lemon juice (ten parts of one organic lemon to one part of warm filtered water) to relieve the pressure. The lemon juice solution creates an osmotic effect by yinnising the area, thus assisting the outflow of the aqueous humour, thus reducing the pressure.

Retinal Detachment

This is a yin characteristic with a focal loss of vision when the retina, which is the membrane that receives the light at the back of the eye, loosens or separates. This condition allows the vitreous fluid to fill the sub retinal space thus separating the retina from its proper place. The sensory layers of the retina progressively pull away from the pigmented epithelium due to the continued yin condition of the individual. Separation may occur suddenly or may develop slowly over years. Medical remedies include photo coagulation by laser or cryothermy, both burn or freeze, respectively, the tear margins and promote inflammation and scarring to seal the hole or the tear.

If the detachment is not serious one can encourage the eye to reform naturally, allowing a holistic process of healing to take place by reducing yin intake as per the yin yang diet. Taking care to reduce 'clean' liquid to ½ - ¾ of a litre a day. To help cure this ailment one can include in the prescribed amount of liquid, infusions of natural diuretics like dandelion, nettle, burdock and fennel. Avoiding yin foods such as sugar, fruit, alcohol, salads, spices etc.. Ginseng will also help the body to yangise thus reducing the eye detachment.

Macular Degeneration

The macular is a small area in the centre of the retina about the size of this 'O', responsible for acute central vision used for reading, facial recognition, driving, watching TV or fine work such as a jeweller etc.. This area degenerates creating fuzzy or blurred vision. This is caused by excesses of yang and yin foods:- such industrialised foods with chemical additives at the beginning or at the end of the food chain, including dairy products, red meat, salt, alcohol, spices, tropical fruits, tomatoes, potatoes etc. (*See* Yin Yang Diet). Activities including smoking and excess VDU use will assist the degeneration of the macular. Balancing diet and eye exercises will allow this area to repair itself or stop the degeneration especially in older people.

Eye Exercise and Massage

I pointed out at the beginning of this section that most of Western science has not yet accepted the fact that chi exists. Most medical cures are symptomatic, the prescribed drugs and their side effects are directed at symptoms, ignoring the cause. Exercise, diet, environment and the condition of the soul all effect the internal energy. When the chi of a person is harmonious, the energy of the mind and body will be balanced, 'dis-ease' occurring when the chi is either too yin or too yang. When the latter three of the above conditions are resolved, correct exercise will encourage the chi to flow and balance more readily. This also applies to the eyes. The flow of blood and its healing properties are encouraged and supported by harmonious chi flow. The following eye exercises will assist all the above complaints to heal by balancing the energy of the organs and the eyes themselves.

After completing 1) from Part 3 do the following as often as is convenient, preferably every morning when chi is more yang:

a) Do each of the following four times with closed lids:-
~~ circle the eyes in a clockwise and anti-clockwise circle (*fig.7a*); ~~ point eyes upward and downward and to left and right in (+)(*fig.7b*);
~~ move the eyes in a diagonal fashion (X) (*fig.7c*);
~~ direct eyes around an imagined horizontal figure of eight (∞). (*fig.7d*)

b) Focus on near and far objects.

c) Take the third finger of both hands and simultaneously, massage gently eight times each of the following acupoints. Firstly the inner part of the eye socket where the corner of the eye meets the nose at (UB.1). Then secondly at the hollow of the temple just behind the external angle of the eye (GB.1) on the side of the head. Then with a curled second finger supported by the first finger (thumb) trace lightly from (UB.1) over the upper and lower part of the closed eyes, in a gentle stroking fashion, away from the eye over the temple (GB.1) along to the ear.(*fig.7e*).

d) After doing 1) from Part 3, use the first half of the micro-cosmic orbit from 2) which is to take the chi up over the head to the yintang (GV25.5) at the third eye point, between the eyes on an in breath. Then on the out breath, imagine the chi to circle each eye, four times (left eye clockwise and right eye anti-clockwise, *See* 1b Part 3.). Then on the in breath, reverse the flow of the visualised chi four times. Lastly to complete the cycle, exhale gently through the nose, imagining any 'dead' energy, being expelled by the breath through the nose. Repeat the complete cycle four times. (*fig.7f*).

e) This closing exercise can be done at any time to relieve eye strain or help healing as it settles the chi in the area of the eyes. Rub the palms of the hands vigorously to produce friction chi then place the cupped palms gently over each eye whilst breathing naturally and repeat as often as is comfortable. One should do this closing exercise, a minimum of four times to finish off any eye exercises.

Always check with a medical practitioner if you are going to take herbal remedies whilst taking prescribed medicines.

Fainting - Syncope - Seizures - Epilepsy

All are varying degrees of the same syndrome, if not directly caused by damage to the brain due to a serious trauma from a blow to the head or a brain tumour. These can be diagnosed with magnetic resonance scanning etc., being desirable in order to find any physical cause. For example brain tumours can be caused by excess use of mobile phones which in turn can cause an epileptic fit by the pressure on the brain. This may need surgery as well as a complete change of lifestyle and diet. (*See* Stress Section).

Generally, seizures are a state of becoming unconscious, which is where the ego consciousness loses its grip on conscious control. Consciousness being subdued because an unconscious factor has reached a greater energy level than the conscious charge of the ego. Hence the fainting or seizure takes place. In other words the ego is overwhelmed by the unconscious invasion for whatever reason, depending very much on the individual.

I am

The ego is a complex, a coming together, of associations built up over the maturing years, determined by inheritance, race, culture, environment and so forth. The ego forms an actual cohesive 'I am' at around seven years of age, depending on the child. Before this time, children tend to say 'we' as they identify their consciousness collectively with their parents and environment. The outward facing part of the ego is the tool which enables an individual to make sense of and deal with the outside world. In moments of stress a person can lose the cohesion of the ego conscious complex and it is split apart temporarily. In extreme cases, it can be more lasting as in severe schizophrenia. The ego complex is two headed, having an inner looking aspect as well as the more accepted outer face. It is the filter which sorts out the data it receives on its bi-directional, reflective capability. (For further detail on the ego complex, refer to my book ***Time for a Change***)

Seizures occur when this centre of consciousness is scattered by something that is too strong for it to cope with. Its cohesive light is diminished or separated. This allows the unconscious contents to break through. Fainting, syncope, seizure and epilepsy are terms that describe different levels of the severity of an unconscious possession. Epilepsy is derived from the word 'to seize or take hold of' and faint means weak and so forth.

General epilepsy is described by medical science as an uncontrolled electrical charge from the nerve cells of the surface of the brain and so diagnosed as a biological disorder. This premise assumes that there is no other function besides a set of chemical and biological reactions that run the body. Yet it is an empirical truth that there is an internal energy of the organism which exists. Over two thirds of the world accept this fact. The Chinese call this energy chi (*See* Part 3) which is an electrical force that circulates and supports the mind and body and when the energy is no longer, the person is no longer.

Kirlian Photography

The effects of the chi field can be captured by 'Kirlian' Photography where an imprint of the residue of the Electro-magnetic fields caused by the meridians and their confluences can be

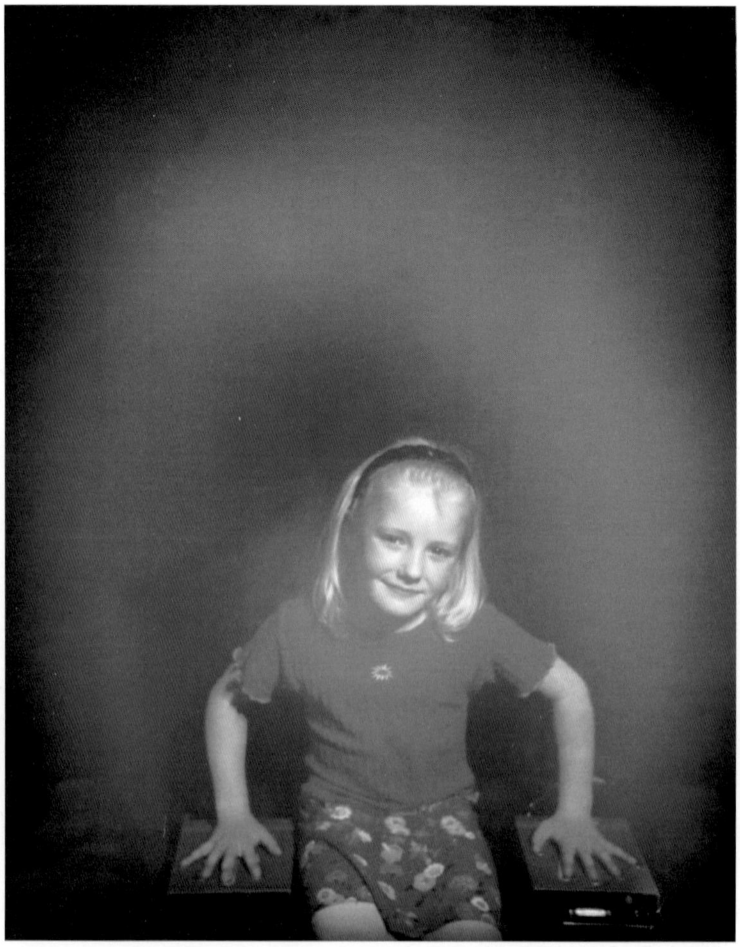

Figure 8: A Kirlian photograph of my daughter, Melissa and her golden aura taken at the Mind Body Spirit Festival, London, 1996. The energy fields are now used in medical research and in defense applications.

observed in photographic form. Kirlian photography since its discovery in 1939, is reasonably well known for depicting this 'aura'. It only emanates from live humans and plants, this energy field ceasing after death. Less well known is that the Russian inventor and electrician, Semyon Davidovich Kirlian and a surgeon Dr. Kuzmich Gaikin who came across acupuncture during his military service in China. Dr Gaikin studied 'Kirlian photographs' of the body and noticed that there were loci which featured in a lighter spectrum seeming to tally with the acupuncture points that the Chinese had mapped out in 2400.BC. (Psychic Discoveries Behind the Iron Curtain by Sheila Ostrander & Lynn Shroeder Prentice-Hall, Inc.). It is claimed by some alternative healers, that the colour and shape of these auras are a guide as to the state of the health and well being of an individual. (*fig.8*)

The various biological reactions are the superficial effects of this energy, which is affected by outer as well as inner stimuli, which in the case of epilepsy can be registered by the electroencephalograph, ECG. The ECG detects and records the electrical activity in the brain by registering potential differences between electrodes placed on the scalp, arising as a result of 'feeble currents' in the brain.

This is proved by the way dogs can sense in advance a seizure and warn their owners.

The Lie Detector

This type of technology was pioneered in 1904 by Professor Jung who was aware of the internal energy of the body when he invented the 'lie detector'. He originally designed this method of measurement to detect the valency of the feeling tone of unconscious complexes. He noted that the greater the resistance on the skin of the patient, the more problematic and resistant was the underlying complex, and so forth. This ability of the brain to emit electrical impulses is exploited in sophisticated fighter aircraft where the brain waves of the pilot are programmed into the plane's computers, in order to speed up pilot to aircraft responses. Telepathy, telekinesis and so forth exploit this ability of the brain to emit signals, by way of its energy waves. This can be compared to the invisible signals of a mobile phone network. Only coherent and identifiable, if one can tune to the correct frequency with the right equipment, to extract the messages from the ether. Intuitive people have this talent.

Crime and Soul

Jung cites a case in an essay on 'Crime and the Soul' in volume eighteen, paragraphs 800-821 from his Collected Works. Here a young boy of twelve is sited as having epileptic fits. Jung discovered the fits were an alternative way for the young boy to replace his morbid moods, fits of depression, aggressive and unconventional behaviour such as running to the cellar and hiding. The parents had observed this behaviour from the age of six. Dr Jung uncovered, after patiently gaining the confidence of the young boy that at the age of six he had been gripped by an inner terror when a man appeared before him asking him to take a sin from him. This apparition terrified the boy because the man, who had a pointed beard wanted him take hold of the sin of murder.

At the age of nine he threw a pair of scissors at his sister which nearly killed her. The force of the throw was such, that he embedded the blades into her skull. The attacks of fear continued to happen to the poor boy, for three years. The mystery man being replaced gradually by a veiled figure of a nursing nun who later became unveiled, only to expose her frightening deathlike pallor underneath. This female spectre continued until the age of twelve, when he was diagnosed as having epilepsy.

The two apparitions were archetypes, the first of which was the malevolent shadow aspect of the boy's psyche manifested by the intimidating man with a pointed beard. Whereas the nun, although not apparently benevolent represented the protective anima, giving rise to the slow process of the ensuing disease. This became the boy's inner method of dealing with this archetypal malice against his sister, being his psyche's way of subduing his violent feelings. The violence, not the moods, stopped after the incident with his sister, being replaced progressively by the onslaught of the epileptic fits.

Energy and The Psyche

As Jung pointed out again and again, if an unconscious source of a disturbance is brought to light, a healing process takes place. Thus the psyche is united and not split, creating a whole. Summed up in his quote, "*The body is the mere visibility of the soul and the soul is the psychological experience of the body*".

This exceptional case, highlights the ability of the psyche to repress or change the conscious state, because of a truth that is too much for the ego consciousness to bear. So, a failsafe mechanism comes into being, as a compensation, to subdue or manipulate the effect of an inner or outer happening.

Fainting is a similar device, where the psyche has confronted an event too charged for the individual to remain conscious, so it shuts off as a defence mechanism. A less evident yet equally disturbing seizure is the symptom of writer's cramp where a person wants to pursue their writing, but is prevented by a blank. Here an unconscious part of the psyche inhibits the creative writing to continue. A similar type of symptom is common amongst successful sports people, where they lose their ability to perform for no apparent physical reason. The real resolve is honest and careful reflection of the psyche which would reveal the underlying cause. Starting as ever by looking into one's soul by way of dreams.

Dream Cure

If any seizures great or small are happening a lot and there is no diagnosed brain damage, the sufferer must do some soul searching to discover the cause. A good place to begin is to take heed of dreams which are a medium for the unconscious contents to permeate into consciousness, by way of the inward looking part of the ego. Dreams are an in built, automatic system of compensation, naturally available in all psyches. Therefore their contents will advise or point out the area of concern, albeit in a symbolic language. This unique and unbiased medium can give free and objective advice, any night. Just like any teacher or friend one must be open and turn an acceptable face towards the unconsciousness to fully benefit from its wisdom. Otherwise we inevitably meet our unconscious as fate. Fate becoming, the avoidable outer half, of the neglected inner split.

I suggest the salient works on dreams by Carl Jung to begin with and or any of the books by Dr. Marie-Louise Von Franz. These will help explain the symbols and the archetypes which although universal are imparted in an individual manner to each person as each psyche is unique. Dream dictionaries and books, which attribute specific meaning to certain criteria in a dogmatic way, should be avoided as they describe misleading stereotypes. Similar to the blanket horoscopes peddled in the media, which cannot possibly apply to each and every individual, from the same sign of the zodiac throughout the world. Dreams have a personal psychic language relating to the sex, age and culture etc. of an individual. For example a male asthmatic may dream of cat which could represent a fear of an allergic reaction or a disturbance in his feminine aspect. Whereas for a female cat lover, a similar dream of a psychic feline could be a positive feeling and a sign of well being, and so forth.

Diet

Despite the inner causes of a seizure, people of a more yin constitution, including pregnant women and people with hypotension etc. seem to be more prone to mild or serious seizures or fainting. Therefore the yin yang diet, being energy balanced, will greatly assist the process of healing. Also seizures can be physically added to by an extreme yang diet, consisting of high salt intake and animal protein, because this creates an overly constricting or yang condition including high blood pressure. The yin yang diet is safe for both categories.

The yin individuals should avoid the yin substances such as sugar and its by products, alcohol, drugs, aspirins, chemical additives, coffee, fruit and fruit juice, spices and dairy food. All of which cause expansion and yinisation of the organism. Ensuring to increase yang food of organic grains and the more root vegetables.

Whereas someone with a yang constitution must eat little or no salt or salty by products, chemical food additives, dairy food, animal protein or fish and consume more leafy green vegetables and soft cooked grains, pasta etc. preferably stir-fried or quickly cooked.

Herbs that can ease seizures are skullcap, mistletoe, vervain, valerian, St. John's Wort and passionflower.

Exercise and Massage

Tai Chi Chuan, Chi Kung, Yoga and light exercise in natural environments will centre the psyche and internal energy. Thus relieving the outer symptoms of seizures. If the causes are exacerbated by yang elements of food, stress and a tendency to hypertension (high blood pressure), the person should do the Chi Kungs, 1), 2) & 3), from Part 3, preferably early mornings. Then sit quietly with hands placed over the abdomen as in 1) in a meditative manner doing 1), focusing the mind on the Tan Tien at the abdomen (CV.6 - *fig.14*) for a comfortable period. This lowers the chi energy in the upper body and head and will help to reduce blood pressure.

If one is more yin and has tendency to hypotension (low blood pressure) perform 1), 2) & 3), in the early morning then do the first part of 2) by taking the chi up over the head to the Yintang (GV24.5) and focusing the mind's eye at that point whilst breathing as in 1).

To help restore a person who has suffered a seizure, for whatever reason, there is usually a disturbance of chi in the 'Governing Vessel'. A disruption of energy in this channel that feeds chi to the brain is the energetic cause of the seizure. This altered state can be triggered by an excess of drugs, alcohol, diet, epilepsy or emotional distress. The symptoms are loss of memory, a slowing down of brain function, light-headedness, blurred vision, eyes rolling back, unstable posture, especially the neck and head, tongue becoming loose, mouth opening, distorted speech, nausea etc.. These symptoms are produced, for whatever underlying reason, by the interference of the chi flow up to the head and around the brain by way of the Governing Vessel. An effective way to help restore the chi flow and bring a person round from a mild seizure is, to first place the person in the recovery position. Then gently stimulate the top lip at the point Renzhong/Yinjiao (GV.26/GV.28 - *fig.14*) in a clockwise fashion with the thumb or index finger lightly. At the same time, gently massaging the nape of the neck at the Jamen Gate (GV.15), at the base of the hairline with the fingers of the free hand. When a clear flow of chi is restored along the meridian, the faculties return.

Always check with a medical practitioner if you are going to take herbal remedies whilst taking prescribed medicines.

Heart, Circulatory Problems and Blood Pressure

The heart according to the Huang Ti Nei Ching, The Yellow Emperor's Treatise on Internal Medicine from ancient China written c. 2500 BC., is the organ of circulation nestled into the centre of the chest with the lungs acting as 'wings' inter relating with the 'Yi', translating as mind, intention or idea. The later Taoist alchemists also considered circulation and consciousness to be connected, associating to both the same reverential attribute of the element Fire, Li of the Five Elements and the Hexagram Fire from the I Ching. Another virtue given to the combination of the heart and the mind was its hermetic ability to transform the primal essence of the kidney into spirit through meditation. Attributing to the heart an inner essence of fire and consciousness.

The Heart Chakra

Various associations granted to the heart, whether true or false, are not exclusive to China being common to all cultures. In Kundalini Yoga the heart chakra of ansata represents the Brahmin element of Air. This is a chakra where consciousness has been elevated from the lower primordial chakras of Earth, Water and Fire respectively. Both East and West allocate the heart as the symbolic centre of love and in other instances courage, for example Richard the Lion Heart. In the past, tribal warriors would cut out and even eat the heart of their enemy to absorb the latent potential of their defeated foe. In Traditional Chinese Medicine the heart besides being connected to consciousness, the soul, the summer, gold, midday and the emotion of joy, is also a part of the anatomy that circulates the blood and so forth. Over a thousand years ago Chinese surgeons used to practice various forms of heart surgery under anaesthesia, only to discover, it was more efficient to heal the whole patient, than trying to cure just one component of the organism, realising that all parts were inter-dependent. It took the Western science a further four thousand years to accept the heart as a form of crude pump. This discovery was attributed to William Harvey (1578-1637) physician to James I and Charles I of England. He studied in Padua, Italy where he learned of the valves in the veins. Thereafter he concluded that the heart pumped blood out through the arteries and back through the veins.

The Heart and Mind

Tai Chi Masters reputedly could control their heartbeat slowing it down to limit the consumption of their chi, internal energy, because they considered the heart to be fired by the inner breath of chi which flows through the various meridians of the body. My first encounter with this phenomenon was in the 1960's, when I saw a French film documentary about a French yogi in Paris. Whilst being closely observed by medical doctors, with journalists in attendance, he was able to control and slow his heart beat progressively, confirmed and monitored by an electrocardiograph, until it stopped for about a ten seconds. Whilst still lying down and being checked all the time by doctors, his heartbeat returned to normal, without any ill effects.

Anyone who has experienced the pleasure of love will also know that this all too human factor of our being can put an actual feeling of a burden on the heart by the emotions of pain, distress and joy. These are experienced as actual sensations in the chest, even when there are no physical symptoms. Whereas a heavy heart and grief can also be felt as a physical pressure on the body, eulogised by poets expressing these heart-felt emotions in their poetry. People can suffer or die of broken hearts. The examples of non-physical symptoms attached to the heart are endless. As well as its other associations, such as the heart being a metaphor for a centre, like in the saying, 'getting down to the heart of the matter'. To truly absorb something one has to learn it by heart.

It is very clear that human beings, throughout history, have quite rightly attributed emotional feelings to the heart, which unfortunately is now scientifically considered simply a pump. Yet doctors know that stress on its own can adversely effect the performance of the heart, accepting the connection between emotional instability and the heart as well as, the purely physical deterioration due to poor diet, stress, lack of exercise, obesity and smoking etc..

Even today's scientists admit that they do not know how the heart actually maintains its rhythm, although in maturity, it becomes connected to the nervous system. In the womb, the heart of the embryo initially is not joined to any nerve fibres, despite maintaining an independent, yet clearly measurable cardiac pulsation. Additionally this phenomenon has been observed outside the organism in the laboratory. Where fragments of cardiac tissue continue to contract rhythmically on their own without any connection or outside stimulus. Furthermore there is no gradation in degree of contraction of the muscle fibres of the heart in situ, which would be the norm if it were under direct nervous control.

The Fire of the Heart

Therefore the heart does have an inner fire and a form of consciousness of its own. It seems that the Chinese doctors from the past were right when they determined that the heart was attached to the mind, fuelled by the internal energy. This perspective would explain many of the so called mysteries surrounding this marvellous pump, such as the absence of an orthodox medical reason for the pains in the arms which accompany heart attacks. This is easily explained by Complementary Medicine because the meridian that controls the heart energy or chi runs up and down each arm. Due to pressure on medical services paramedics always ask a potential heart attack patient if he or she has pains in the chest and the arms in order to focus and speed up diagnosis.

The Mind and Memory of The Heart

Cellular memory is now an accepted medical fact where transplant patients have memories that can only be attributed to the psyche of the donor. This tale from a Channel 4 UK documentary, concerns an English man in his fifties who received a heart transplant. On the way home from hospital, when he entered the car he was overcome with extreme sadness, causing him to cry then he experienced, in his mind's eye an accident, heard the screech of tyres and the smell of fuel and burning. He thought little of it, putting it down to patient fear after being enclosed for six weeks in hospital. Then, for the first time in his life he started listening to classical music. After a whole host of such novel interests that came from nowhere he and his wife started to hear rumours of this phenomenon concerning transplant patients with similar incidents.

He then managed to contact through the hospital the donor's family, whereupon he discovered that he had been given the heart of a young man who had died in a car accident who loved classical music. So the heart of the young man in his last seconds had registered his grief at the loss of his own life and young family as well as passing on personal traits. For further information - *Gary E Swartz, Professor of Psychology, Surgery, Medicine, Neurology and Psychiatry University of Arizona, USA.*

The documentary then showed tests carried out at University College London where volunteers had their hearts and minds monitored simultaneously. Whether shown distressing or pleasurable material the hearts of the volunteers picked up the emotion first before the brain.

The following are all caused by excesses of yin and yang foodstuffs, lifestyle and stress.

Arteriosclerosis and Atherosclerosis

Before the rampant consumer society arteriosclerosis (a more yang complaint) was the most common arterial disease which targeted mainly the old. Now, however it is prevalent in all ages and sexes. It is a hardening of the arteries normally preceded by atherosclerosis which is when fatty deposits line the inner walls of the arteries. The deposits reduce the normal flow of blood through the arteries putting undue pressure on the heart. Cholesterol is associated to these fatty substances and as the atherosclerosis progresses; calcium is deposited creating a plaque. Scar tissue develops causing the walls to loose their elasticity. Arteriosclerosis can affect any or all the arteries of the body and if the blood vessels that feed the heart become clogged it can result in the very painful disease called:

Angina Pectoris

This is a yang condition, characterised by severe pains in the chest and arms. Angina is caused by cardiac ischemia (yang) which is an insufficient blood flow through the coronary arteries of the heart musculature due to plaque deposits in the coronary arteries. One medical procedure is to try and open the closed artery with 'balloon angioplasty'. A catheter is manoeuvred to the offending blockage by way of the femoral artery in the leg, right up the body, through the aorta at the apex of the heart, where a surgical 'balloon' is inserted and inflated to free the obstruction by flattening the plaque.

If this fails a Coronary Bypass can be the next surgical procedure to prevent a Heart Attack, by grafting veins from the legs to bypass the diseased artery of the heart. Arteriosclerosis can precipitate a clot known as a thrombus where the plaque breaks off causing a blockage further on. If serious enough, it will give rise to a thrombosis:

Coronary Thrombosis

This is also a yang condition, also a localised dilation of an artery called an Aneurysm may also develop. A simple Complementary Medicine test to see if the arteries have hardened is to put both hands together prayer fashion. Unless physically damaged, one takes into account the flexibility of the wrist, which should fairly easily make a ninety degree angle between the back of the hand and the wrist. The degree of the angle and difficulty will indicate the relative hardening.

Strokes

These are usually caused by arterial blockage provoked by either a Thrombosis or an Embolism (extreme yin or yang). A thrombosis involves atherosclerotic plaque, in one or more of the four main arteries leading to the brain. As these arteries become narrowed, a potential stroke victim often experiences recurrent warnings of transient paralysis. Usually experienced in one arm or leg or on one side of the face, or impaired speech, vision, or other motor functions. At this stage, deposits in the linings of the cerebral arteries can often be treated by surgery, including laser surgery and microsurgical bypass of blockages.

Strokes can also be caused by a haemorraging in the brain, when these blood vessels become yin, thus weak.

Embolism

This occurs when a cerebral artery suddenly becomes blocked by material coming from another part of the bloodstream. These solid masses, or emboli, often form as clots in a diseased or malfunctioning heart, but can also come from dislodged fragments of atherosclerotic plaque or even an air bubble.

Abnormal Blood Pressure: –

Hypertension

This is a yang condition caused by extremes of yin or yang) is the elevation of arterial blood pressure above the norm of 120/80 for a healthy person in their thirties and is a precursor to many of the conditions mentioned. It is caused by an over consumption of yin dilatory substances:- such as excess fluids, sugary foods, spices, yin drugs, all causing the heart to yinnise and thus work harder, to circulate the blood. Also high blood pressure can be due to excess yang intake such as salt, dairy food, animal protein, which yangises the kidneys creating a pressure build up as the nephrons of the kidney contract reducing blood flow, thus building up pressure in the arteries. Yang drugs, stress, anxiety and hectic lifestyles accompanied by poor eating habits will also cause high blood pressure by tightening the organism, thus restricting circulation. One must be careful also with substances such as ginseng which can raise blood pressure because it stimulates adrenocorticotropic hormone being a very yang herb.

Hypotension

This is a yin complaint, being the opposite where the blood pressure drops below the norm of 120/80 being caused by a yinnising of the body due to excess fluid loss.

Myocardial Infarction

Being a yin complaint, describes when the blood supply to the heart is obstructed caused by an over consumption of yin substances which yinnise or reduce the output of the heart to such a degree that the normal healthy circulatory pressure lowers.

Tachycardia (yang)

This is the term which describes the heart beat when it goes above 100 beats per minute, usually a natural function to increase blood supply during and after exercise, not having an adverse affect in a healthy person. Stress will also cause tachycardia which is a tense yangisation of the body, unnaturally increasing the heart rate to cope with the stress. This can be engendered by adrenaline being pumped into the blood. This yang neurohormone is allied to the internal energy or chi of the organism. When the yang chi of the body is activated, it increases heart rate.

This is yangisation process is exploited in a harmless way in Chi Kung which fires up the chi naturally increasing heart rate but without any physical stress. This makes Chi Kung the most energy efficient cardio-vascular exercise possible, yet without any movement or physical exertion. Tachycardia is also triggered by fear. (*See* Part 3 Chi Kung). Fear is the emotion that is allied to the organ of the kidney in Complementary Medicine. Therefore when this yang energy of the kidney is released unnaturally, by fear or stress, in the old or frail, it can bring on this form of tachycardia causing extreme concern and even leading to heart failure.

Cure and Diet

All the mentioned physical heart and circulatory problems are caused by an excess consumption of extremes of yin and yang food especially fatty foods derived from animal protein, exacerbated by lack of exercise, hectic lifestyle, smoking, pollution and stress. The yin yang diet must be adhered to until all the symptoms are resolved with care taken to balance diet and lifestyle thereafter.

When suffering yang heart complaints, which cause restriction, slightly more yin foods should be carefully consumed. The converse applies to yin heart complaints by consuming a bit more of the yang foods (*See* Yin Yang Diet).

Also one has to balance the amount of Cholesterol, which is a steroid produced and needed by the body to support various tissues and build hormones. Normal levels of the right sort of cholesterol are an essential component of the blood stream, to ensure healthy arteries. There are two types of cholesterol carrying proteins in the blood formed in the liver. Firstly high density lipoproteins, HDL and low-density lipoproteins, LDL. LDL is a major factor of atherosclerosis. Whereas HDL reduces unwanted cholesterol in the bloodstream bringing it back to the liver to be processed. It is considered that high levels of LDL in the blood plasma form the plaque and so increase the risk of heart attacks and heart disease. Organic whole grains, pulses, fruit and vegetables reduce harmful cholesterol levels, but one must follow the seasonal and environmental guidelines of the yin yang diet to guarantee all round balance. Garlic in moderation, some fish oils, cold pressed, organic 'virgin' vegetable oils such as sesame, safflower and olive oils all help to reduce harmful levels of cholesterol. Regular and sensible consumption of oily fish is very beneficial for the circulatory system.

Herbs for The Heart and Circulation

Herbs that are good for the heart and circulation have been known for centuries. A lot of drugs, although based on plant remedies, are usually synthesised making them unnatural, thus losing their integral value. The most well known being digitalis, strengthens the contraction of the heart being a yang herb. Whereas the yin remedy of rutin, a derivative of buckwheat, dilates the system reducing hardening of the arteries, hypertension and unnecessary clotting. The yang inducing Astragalus is used in Chinese Medicine to strengthen the heart. It is better known as locoweed in the cowboy country of the North American prairies where it grows in the wild. If errant hungry livestock overeat this weed, it causes them to become frenzied or extreme yang. Loco is the Spanish for crazy, hence the hybrid word 'loco'weed.

Science has discovered Astragalus to contain selenium which scavenges up the body's, unwanted free radicals. It is an accepted heart tonic in Western herbal medicine as well. The Chinese yin herb, Gingko, is now popular in the West due to its anti-clotting and circulatory enhancing properties. Hawthorn or white thorn is a tried and tested heart restorative and vasodilator which has been used for centuries. These herbs can only be successfully used as tonics for the heart and circulatory system if used correctly and in conjunction with a balanced diet and lifestyle. Always use herbs cautiously as one would a medicine because they only ease the symptoms. For a whole cure the actual causes have to be addressed. The amazing garlic besides being an internal and external bactericide is excellent at promoting a healthy circulatory system even breaking down cholesterol and calcium deposits. But garlic is a yin bulb, so use sparingly. However if required regularly, about one clove a day will keep the doctor away.

Exercise

Learning how to relax by finding one's centre both physically and mentally will greatly ease the pressure on this vital system of circulation. (*See* Stress Section). Tai Chi Chuan, Chi Kung and Yoga less so, can be easily be learnt and practised by any age of person who has suffered heart disease, without any concern. They are tried and tested cardiovascular exercises which heal and strengthen the whole body including the heart and nervous system naturally, without inducing any strain. These type of disciplines can be done in a relaxed manner, when recuperating and even after recent surgery, if feeling well.

Also any gentle movement is beneficial, like walking in the fresh air, ensuring not to enter into any unnecessary physical exertion. But Tai Chi and Chi Kung are especially beneficial and will gently iron out the excess of yin and yang chi in the body, being the energetic causes of the heart problem, however induced. All exercise must be accompanied by a balanced diet after a change in lifestyle. This collective formula will ensure a cure. If any heart disease is caught early enough, a change in diet, exercise and lifestyle can prevent the need for unnecessary medication with all the negative side effects and or surgical intervention.

To relieve hypertension, one can carry out the following exercise at any time for as long as is comfortable, possibly five to ten minutes to begin with. One should sit quietly with hands placed over the abdomen as in 1), from Part 3 on Chi Kung, in a relaxed meditative manner whilst doing 1). All the time keeping a focus of the mind on the Tan Tien at the abdomen (CV.6 - *fig.14*). This mind focusing at the Tan Tien lowers the chi pressure from the upper body and head and so reduces blood pressure.

As well as the chi calming exercise, one can do the following Chi Kungs, 1), 2) & 3), from Part 3. All are very beneficial for the circulatory system and heart, especially if done early morning.

However if one is more yin and has tendency to hypotension perform 1), 2) & 3), in the early morning. Then do the first part of 2), by taking the chi up over the head to the Yintang (GV.25.5 - *fig.14*). Then, whilst focusing the mind's eye at that point on the forehead, continue the reverse breathing as in 1).

Chi Kungs 1) & 2) can be practised before, during or after medical treatment however serious. When one is well on the road to recovery or as a prevention besides 1) & 2), one can do 7) & 8), being specific Chi Kungs to balance the energy of the internal organs, including the heart and circulation.

Summary

The heart beat in modern medicine is extremely well tabulated, but its actual impulse to contract is not understood, whereas in Complementary Medicine the internal energy, the chi, is accepted as the source of its energy supply. Not only stimulating the nerves that control the heart, but also the heart's own autonomous system of the sinoauricular node (SA node). The SA node manages the contraction of the auricles and in turn innervates the lower auriculoventricular node (AV node), being responsible for the action of the muscles of the ventricles. These seemingly independent nodes innervate the four chambers of the heart to contract and expand in order to circulate the blood and nutrients around the body.

It is because chi is the motivator of the heart and linked to the psyche, that stress as well as feelings have an effect on the heart and its circulatory ability. Absent healing where a group of people pray for another who is ill, often is successful. This phenomenon is exploited in Tai Chi Chuan and Chi Kung where the mind is able to connect with the internal energy by visualisation and mind intent. Then the chi can be circulated for benevolent or more rarely malevolent purposes. This is summed up in the Tai Chi Chuan maxim' the mind moves the chi that moves the body. Hypnotists and manipulative persons including politicians, business magnates exploit this ability of the psyche to control others by this way of projecting. However a person can also interfere with his or her own energy circulation albeit in an unconscious manner. For example if a person does not want to do something yet suppresses that fact down into the personal unconsciousness, by self-deception, this negative impulse can appear as fate either in the body manifesting as illness or even an accident. (*See **Time for a Change***).

The Heart of the Matter

In the early 1990's a medical centre in Washington USA, wanted to find out why Italians who drank alcohol, did little or no exercise, often smoked and eat meat, surprisingly suffered little heart trouble. Whereas the non-smoking clean living Washingtonians who jogged, drank little or no alcohol, eating calorie-controlled diets had higher incidents of heart disease.

The conclusion was that these American Italians were happy family orientated people with a high fibre diet of pasta, laced with garlic, olive oil, tomatoes and wine who could laugh stress away, as opposed to the fraught and stressed materialists. However controlled their lifestyles seemed, it did little to alleviate the pressure on their cardio-vascular system.

This is yet another proof that the internal energy of the body is connected to the inner being. So if the psyche is at peace, with the mind and body being at one and relaxed, the condition of the organism will respond accordingly.

The Outer Aspects of the Heart

In Complementary Medicine the relationship of the outer effect of the internal energy manifests itself in the face. It is an instant and useful diagnostic tool. The microcosmic image of heart chi manifests itself in various ways, especially visible in the macrocosm of the face. The form and size of the face being relative to the shape of the heart. A round yang face corresponds to a round yang heart and so forth. Also the four chambers of the heart correlate to the face. If you divide the rough circle of the face into four, the central point being located at the cross section of a horizontal line just below the eyes and the vertical running up through the nose. The top two quadrants of the face, around and over the eyes, depict the relative top two atriums of the heart. The lower two quadrants of the face around the cheeks and jaw are linked to the lower two ventricles.

Discoloration of one or all areas, especially a reddening indicates a corresponding problem in the related area of the heart. If the central tip of the nose has a cleft it shows the heart to be beating irregularly or the presence of murmuring. An enlarged nose will reveal a swollen heart usually due to eating and drinking too much. These superficial, diagnostic techniques can be confirmed by a study of the twelve pulses which indicate the state of the internal organs. The six yin and six yang points are located just below the interior or yin side of the wrist, along the lung meridian.

The Heart and Other Organs

Heart disease can also be effected by the condition of the liver. The liver has many life supporting functions, including being responsible for the retention or digestion of fatty substances. It is also responsible for the production of cholesterol and the quality of the blood in general. This obviously has a direct repercussion on healthy circulation. Yin substances, like alcohol, sugar, spices, yin drugs, and the more yang eggs, fatty substances including dairy foods, all reduce liver function. In Complementary Medicine anger is the negative emotion of the liver. If one suffers anger often, the liver function is lowered. When one rises to anger too much due to stress etc. it will adversely effect the energy and function of the liver.

To prevent and keep the heart, arteries and veins in good order, it is advisable to centre one's lifestyle by avoiding extremes of emotion and foods. Stress is caused by fear which is a loss of soul that can be remedied by seeking the inner helper. (*See* Stress Section)

One should always maintain a diet of organic, natural high fibre foods, low in saturated fat accompanied by plenty of fresh organic vegetables. Preferably a diet consisting of foods that are in season and from the same climatic zone as per the yin yang diet. Especially useful for the heart and circulation is leafy green vegetables and salads from the appropriate season and climate. Avoid spinach as it contains oxalic acid which is a poison. Occasional and sensible alcohol intake if desired will do no great harm, but ensure the alcohol to be clean, uncomplicated and not strong. Beer is too bulky and raises blood pressure. Naturally produced red wine in small quantities, say no more than a glass of wine a day, will keep blood circulation healthy. The virtue of oily fish such as cod, halibut, sardines, herrings, mackerel, natural salmon besides being an excellent source of protein will assist heart and circulation. These coupled with regular non strenuous aerobic exercise particularly disciplines like Tai Chi Chuan, Chi Kung, Yoga, walking, non-strenuous cycling and swimming (preferably in the sea or swimming pools with limited, chemically treated water) and so forth will ensure a smooth trouble free circulation.

Always check with a medical practitioner if you are going to take herbal remedies whilst taking prescribed medicines.

Joint Troubles, Aches and Pains, Gout including the Muscles and Tendons

General aches and pains in the body, even if brought about by exercise or habitual work patterns are caused by the body's inability to ensure muscle and joint maintenance. The internal energy, the chi, that runs the organism, despite being responsible for the well being of the internal organs, senses, microbiological structures such as the immune system and so forth, maintaining the skeletal and muscular structure as well. When the internal energy flow around the body is out of harmony or inhibited, besides creating a variety of disorders as laid out in this book it will cause mild or chronic aches and pains. Therefore such pain is a warning, highlighting an energy imbalance.

The limbs can be compared to the branches of a tree. If a branch is diseased, it can relay to an expert the cause of the trouble. The same is true of the limbs in Complementary Medicine. The energy meridians run to and from the vital organs, out and back from the extremities in the hands, feet and head. This phenomenon is inadvertently acknowledged in science, in the case of amputated limbs. When a limb has been amputated there are so called ghost sensations around the area of the missing limb. These all too real sensations including pain are felt because the internal energy is still travelling along the ghost limb (*See* Eye Section). These meridians allow the organs to breath.

When chi is inhibited, or too yin or yang, the energy flow is reduced around joints and muscles, thus causing the pain to the effected areas. The main reason for these imbalances is poor diet, stress and polluted environments, bad posture, over strenuous exercise, EMF fields and accidental trauma. All of these factors can change or interrupt chi flow.

Martial Pain

This knowledge was exploited by the martial Tai Chi masters who could damage joints, muscles, brain function and the internal organs by striking vital points, (specific acupoints) along the energy channels. These Masters, who only acted in self-defence, would hit certain areas to render limbs useless or create a residual effect in an internal organ. The following anecdote is attributed to the eldest son of the founder of the 'Yang' style of Tai Chi Chuan, Yang Pan Hou (1837-1892), which aptly illustrates this ability. This well to do Tai Chi master was foolishly attacked by three brigands whilst he was anonymously disembarking from a ferry boat. He defended himself by using only three counter moves, to dispatch the miscalculating opportunists into the river. Before leaving the site he told the first thief to come and see him in a week, the second in a month and the last attacker in three months. Due to the power and ease of the Masters defence the brigands realised that he meant what he said. Tai Chi masters were often practicing healers as in this case, because each of the thieves became ill at the specified times. The master had used his knowledge of how and when chi flows to interrupt the cyclical flow in each of the men, hence they fell ill at the appointed time, needing the remedial care of Pan Hou. This is not an isolated story. Despite this martial prowess, Tai Chi has always been used to heal more than to hurt, because to reach such a level these masters realised that such skill was nothing compared to the power of the Universal forces,

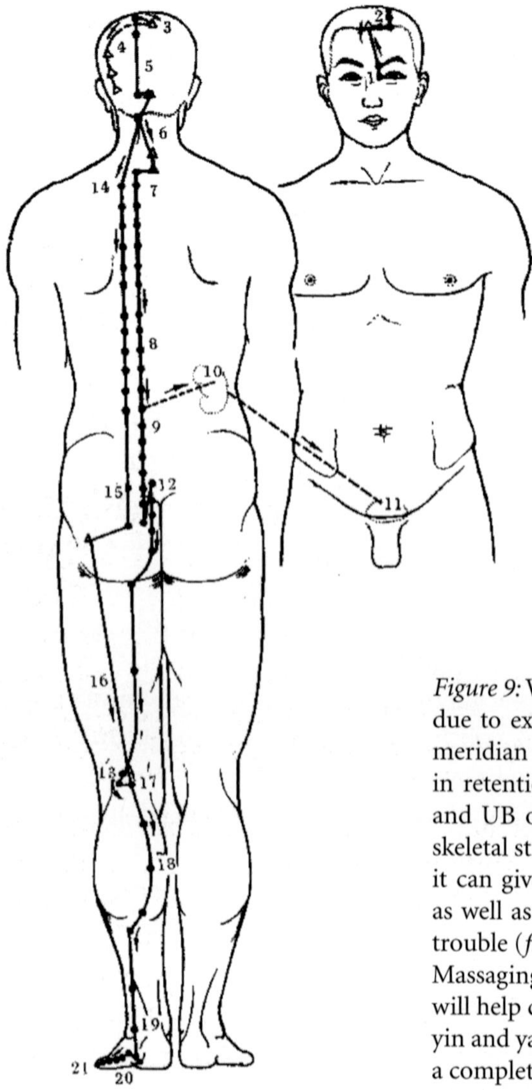

The course of the urinary bladder meridian & the numbered acupoints.

Figure 9: When the internal energy is made 'wet' or too yin, due to excess liquid or toxins, the Urinary Bladder (UB) meridian is disturbed which can cause more fluid and toxin retention creating a vicious cycle. Because the Kidney and UB organs and meridians control the energy of the skeletal structure, when these channels are out of harmony it can give rise to stiffness, aches and pains in the joints, as well as rheumatism, arthritis and Gout including back trouble (*fig. 12*).
Massaging the lower back and along the back UB channel will help clear the symptomatic conditions, but excesses of yin and yang in lifestyle will have to be addressed to ensure a complete cure.

of which human chi is but a minuscule representative, albeit connected.

Tacos, Acupuncture and Anaesthesia

This knowledge of energy flow is applied to heal millions of people daily in China and the Far East. Also acupuncture anaesthesia is employed to isolate nerves in order that surgery may be performed more efficiently, especially on the old and infirm, without loss of consciousness. The internal energy is responsible for feeding the nervous system. When this flow of energy is stimulated by way of certain chi reducing acupoints, it inhibits the normal motor and sensory functions, thus becoming an anaesthetic. Western medicine accepts that there is an electrical charge running through the nervous system and so forth, albeit more superficially than in Complementary Medicine. (*See* Part 3 on chi). The famous Mayo Clinic in Phoenix, Arizona, USA use acupuncture anaesthesia. In 2001 a teacher from California had a worm removed from her brain using acupuncture anaesthesia, in order not to damage brain tissue. She was conscious throughout the successful surgery ensuring that no unnecessary damage occurred during the operation. She ingested the worm on a holiday in Mexico from an undercooked pork taco. It entered her digestive system then lodged itself in the brain. This is common in Latin American Countries and is responsible for many deaths.

The same effect of interfering with chi flow is indirectly achieved, less dramatically than our martial example, by diet, stress, pollution, trauma etc..

Even the more serious nerve diseases are brought about by disharmonious energy flow such as MS, motor neurone disease, muscular dystrophy and so forth. The 'mother load' of chi is passed on by the actual physical mother, so these diseases can be inherited, and in some cases can be reversed, but this will depend on the gravity of the congenital effects on the body's structure and the psyche of the individual concerned.

Water and Pain

The following case is an example of self inflicted pain by excess yin intake caused by the new trend to drink voluminous amounts of water, in order to keep the organism clean. This counter productive medical advice works on the level of preventing a build up of toxins to alleviate kidney failure. This excessive need is engendered by the poor quality of food and drink usually eaten in blind acceptance, due to the popular availability of convenience-industrialised foodstuffs, and also the level pollutants prevalent in our society. Unfortunately this excessive liquid intake has residual consequences which can have long-term effects by over yinnising the body (*See* Part 3).

A fit career orientated man of twenty-eight years of age came to do Tai Chi to cure his 'bad back'. After an initial examination I saw his internal organs and chi flow were in good condition, but his hands were damp and he sweated easily. He informed me that he was advised to drink four litres of water a day to keep his system clean as he did a lot of exercise. Firstly the quality of the water can be detrimental to health on its own as it contains all the harmful residues to be found in tap water, (*See* Part 1). Also the volume of liquid had water logged his kidneys which, just like a sponge, are not effective at cleaning when wet, (*see* Detox section). Also the kidneys, when under duress, reduce their ability to produce internal energy, (*See* Part 2). Secondly the urinary bladder and its meridian were disturbed. Often in such cases the dampness or yinnisation of the small back is caused by excess liquid or for that matter an excess of yin foods (*See* Yin Yang Diet Part 1). The urinary bladder meridian (*fig.10*) runs over the head, down the neck, then descending each side of the back over the kidney area. The chi of this meridian feeds the muscles of the back. When this meridian is damp or yin, the flow of chi to this area is disturbed. This yinnisation will weaken the muscles and render them prone to damage, hence the 'bad back'.

After five weeks of practicing Tai Chi and Chi Kung, reducing liquid and eating a more balanced diet, the lower back trouble of ten years was cured.

The healing process was easily achieved by applying the Complementary Medicine knowledge of internal energy and balancing the energy flow, redressing the imbalance of chi that feeds the muscles and tendons which are conditioned by the chi of the liver and gallbladder. Also harmonising the energy of the bones and skeletal structure, being under the influence of the chi of the kidneys and the urinary bladder.

Chi, Joints and Flow

The quality of the internal energy as well as blood maintains the viscosity of the synovium which is the membrane that surrounds and secretes the fluid that lubricates the cartilage and the joint. The Tai Chi masters proclaim that where chi runs smoothly, blood will do the same. Chi, like blood, has a restricted flow over and around joints due to the natural constrictions around the joint, needed by the complicated mechanics of articulation. Therefore when chi is disrupted, the discomfort will often manifest itself around the joints first. Initially this can effect the principle weight bearing areas like ankles, knees, hips and of course the spine, and or at the extremities where the body mass is narrowed around fingers and toes. Even if the imbalance is long term, resulting in permanent damage to articulation, it can be greatly relieved by the yin yang diet (*See* Part 1) taking into account the highlighted factors in the following Cure section, as well as the suggested exercises from this section.

Therefore depending on age, activity and the condition of the salient organ energy, the level of aches and pains are the result of the deficiency or imbalance of chi. This deficiency can inhibit the performance of a sports superstar or the person indulging in any leisure sport activity like golf, squash, horse-riding, tennis, football and so forth.

Arthritis

Arthritis is a disease of a joint from the Gr. '*Arthron*' + '*Itis*', being the suffix meaning disease. This is a collective medical term covering more than a hundred different types. Arthritis can cause serious disability in many people which has two main areas that I shall cover here, but as all are caused by chi imbalance, brought about by overly yin or yang energy causes. However the following cures can be adapted to heal any of them. Firstly the most common being the degenerative joint disease of osteoarthritis which is non-inflammatory and more yang, and secondly rheumatoid arthritis, where the joints become inflamed and yin.

Osteoarthritis

Statistics show that osteoarthritis usually affects people who are over thirty-five years of age. Sometimes it can begin at an earlier age because of joint injury or overuse. Men and women are affected equally before the age of fifty-five, but there is a higher incidence of osteoarthritis in women over fifty five. Ninety percent of people over sixty show some signs of osteoarthritis. When the cause of osteoarthritis is 'medically' unknown, it is called primary osteoarthritis. When the cause is known, such as injury, and repeated use of the joints (such as the knees, ankles, wrists, elbows, etc.) of sports people, it is called secondary osteoarthritis.

Osteoarthritis destroys the joint cartilage of the major weight-bearing joints of the hips, knees, and spinal column. The disease usually affects only one or two joints. With osteoarthritis, the cartilage of the joints gradually wears away with weight bearing and movement in the joint. As the disease progresses, so much of the cartilage is destroyed that the bone ends begin to rub against each other. Bony spurs develop around the joint, and pain and inflammation result.

Osteoarthritis is not only the most common type of arthritis, it is also the most easily managed. Osteoarthritis is diagnosed, based on the patient's medical history, a physical examination to determine which joints are affected, alongside blood tests, and x-rays. A sample of synovial fluid from the affected joint may also be taken. The main symptom of osteoarthritis is restricted motion in the joint, along with a deep, aching pain during movement and at night, aggravated by joint deformity

Many Western Causes, yet Simply a Yin and Yang Cure

Osteoarthritis and rheumatoid arthritis are caused for a variety of reasons in Western Medicine, over two hundred, but the causes are more simply categorised, by Complementary Medicine, into two categories. Firstly there are the excesses of 'yang' foods like meat, eggs, and salt and salty foods, foods with a high mineral content including the calcium rich dairy foods. These yang extremes are often excessively balanced by, or simply an indulgence in an over consumption of 'yin' substances such as excess fluids in the form of beer, tea and coffee, soft drinks and or spices, tropical fruit, especially citrus fruit, fruit juice, vinegar, aromatic herbs, tomatoes, and exotic vegetables and sugar by-products including chocolate and confection, especially ice cream and cold desserts etc.. Simply yin foods dilate the body, whereas yang contracts whether in the joints, muscles or any body tissue. Yin Yang follows Universal law.

Thus the extremes of yin and yang cause the body to react where there is a weakness in this case, the joints. Each person is different and the causes and effects are unique to each individual even though the symptoms can be the same.

Rheumatoid Arthritis

Statistically rheumatoid arthritis is a chronic disease that can affect children between eight and fifteen years of age and adults between twenty and fifty five years of age. It rarely occurs in those over fifty five. It has a tendency to run in families due to similar diet and lifestyle patterns. However seventy percent of the people affected are over thirty years of age.

Rheumatoid arthritis affects the smaller, more yang compact joints of the hands, wrists, feet, and ankles before it affects joints such as the hips, knees, and elbows. The disease is symmetric and bilateral, meaning that it affects the same joints on both sides of the body because the energy meridians also run in this manner.

Rheumatoid arthritis affects the synovium (synovial membrane), the lining of the joints, which becomes inflamed (red, swollen, painful, and warm). The synovium secretes more fluid, making the joint more swollen. Later, the cartilage also becomes involved and eventually becomes rough and pitted. Ligaments and tendons also become inflamed, scarred, and shortened by the disease, contributing to the deformities often noticed in the hands and wrists of people with rheumatoid arthritis. It is also exacerbated by the sufferer's own immune system which can attack the inflamed joint. This is usually caused by an excess of yin or yang substances. Yang chi defends the organism whereas yin chi attacks.

Gout

Gout is where Uric Acid is in such excess that it deposits painfully around joints, however this method will cure Gout and it's symptoms.

Cure

Although the symptoms are different, osteoarthritis and rheumatoid arthritis are in fact chi imbalance of the internal organs of the liver/GB and kidneys/UB. This also applies to the everyday aches and pains which will benefit greatly from balancing diet as well as exercise. This is evident from my mentioned case history. They are all caused by excesses of yin and yang substances and lifestyle. These problems will equally effect sports persons who have unbalanced diets, due to the interference of correct energy flow, exacerbated by more wear and tear. Therefore, whether the damage is caused by exercise, excesses in lifestyle or simply old age, the cure is the same, but relative depending on the amount of damage already incurred.

The energy producing organs of the kidneys operate more efficiently when they are in a balanced yang state so liquid intake should be uncomplicated and moderate ½ - 1 litre a day, depending on activity and fluid loss. (*See* Diet Section).

The ear is the sense organ in Complementary Medicine attributed to the kidneys being about the same shape and size also indicating the condition of these hard working organs, when overly red, yang, can indicate kidney infection and or too much salt and animal protein. In acupuncture the ear is a curled up microcosm of the whole body, being an upside down image of our foetal origins with the head sited at the earlobe and the upper tip of the ear corresponding to the lower extremities of the body and the limbs. The ears in part or whole can be stimulated to animate the chi of the corresponding parts of the body.

Whereas the liver oversees the energy of the muscles and tendons needing similar attention. An excellent time for everybody to detoxify the liver, is around Mardi Gras, as the name implies being 'Fat Tuesday', so fatty foods or negative 'liver' foods should be eaten for the last time as Winter closes, then given up until the next cold season. Fat and oils were eaten as fuel for the winter. Although it is still a sensible time to purge the liver, the types of food are obviously different because these customs evolved prior to supermarkets and central heating. But Mardi Gras coincides with Complementary Medicine when liver energy is revitalised in the yearly cycle around spring.

Liverish people do not like wind or draughts as these attack liver chi and a good tip is to be near plants and wood of all kinds as these help reinforce liver energy in or out of the house. When these organs are under stress, one will be angry and bilious but when they are harmonious, one retains the useful and necessary opposite emotion in Complementary Medicine of willpower. Thus relieving the general lethargic feeling that these organs can impart when under par. The replenishing chi circulates through the liver and gall bladder from 11.00pm - 1.00am and 1.00am - 3.00am respectively (GMT UK or local solar time). Therefore try to retire before these times and eat lightly, preferably at least three hours before sleep. Otherwise liver chi is depleted unnecessarily.

Diet

Firstly one must follow a balanced organic grain vegan diet excluding all animal protein including dairy food and seafood avoiding all excesses of yang and yin (*See* Part 1, Yin Yang Diet). Keep pure fluids to a minimum.

The diet should consist of 60% yang foods comprising of 'dry' cooked whole cereal grains,

(*See* Yin Yang Diet, Part 1), 20% pulses, 10% yang vegetables, 5% indigenous fruit in season (not acidic), 5% liquid intake (½ - 1 litre) in the form of pure uncomplicated fluids including, filtered water, herb teas (*See below*), exclude all regular coffee or tea, diet and soft drinks etc.. Avoid all dairy foods (cheese, milk, butter and eggs), spices, junk food and particularly food that have additives, preservatives, colouring and so forth. Keep seasoning to a minimum especially salt, preferably use sesame salt and with small amounts of garlic to boost circulation and the immune system. (*See* Yin Yang Diet). The yang part of the diet should be from organic quality grain foods including mainly organic brown rice and buckwheat which are excellent for the digestion and circulation, but a variety of organic whole grain foods and their derivatives are acceptable including millet, cous cous, bulgur, barley, corn, oats, rye, buckwheat and buckwheat noodles and pasta. Try to reduce yeasted whole wheat breads to a minimum; it is preferable to eat the unleavened breads, including chapatis and so forth, until the system ameliorates. One can add organic miso paste to dishes or in soups, or taken as a drink in the morning, by dissolving one teaspoonful of organic miso paste in boiled filtered, but not hot water. The pulses and beans that are good for kidneys are the kidney beans, aduki beans and mung beans. Organic vegetables like carrots, celery, turnips, swede, cauliflower, beans, broccoli, leeks, onions, fennel, chicory, celery, artichokes, radishes, onions and non acidic greens are preferable. Avoid all acidic foods and citrus fruits, tomatoes and their by-products, spinach, eggplant, aubergine and potatoes. Depending on taste cook foods simply like 'stir frying' so as not to waste the nutritional benefits. One can adopt vegan recipes, ensuring to keep to the above balance of yang to yin foods because some vegan diets are far too yin and contain exotic or taboo foods. The body vibrates at a certain yin or yang pitch depending on climate and season. Especially when ill, foodstuffs must be from the same climate and season where the person habitually lives in order to create a harmonious balance of internal and external factors.

Herbs and Plants

These can be beneficial for the kidneys including fennel, parsley, chervil, tarragon, sage, burdock, bladderwort, dandelion and nettle, taken as infusions. Herbs which help the liver are, rosemary, thyme, chervil, celery, tarragon, chive, fennel, cumin, capers, nutmeg, clove, horseradish, wild thyme (serpolet), saffron, extract of artichoke and dandelion. Milk thistle is now generally available from health food stores in capsules and preferably tinctures, being useful for detoxifying the liver.

Drinks which help detox the liver and gall bladder are decoctions of rosemary, thyme, mint, meadowsweet, and camomile, being also tonifying.

Remember herbs are like medicines and over use will reduce their efficacy. So try various ones for limited periods to find out the most suitable.

Massage

First thing after rising in the morning:-

1) Gently tap the lower back over the kidney area with lightly clenched fists being very beneficial because it will stimulate 'kidney' chi.

2) Rub, in a stroking motion, both hands down the outside (yang) of the legs and then back up towards the body on the inside (yin) of the legs, then with one hand rub, in a stroking motion outward away from the body along the outside of the arm (yang) and back up towards the body on the inside of the arm.

3) Rub the ears gently forwards and backwards with the fingers, this will help wake up the kidneys and their chi in the morning.

4) K1, being the start of the kidney acupuncture meridian, which is in the centre of the pad of the feet can be stimulated by hand massage etc. or with a lighted moxa herb bundle or even an incense stick.

Also to alleviate lower back trouble, one can energise and free the area by gently rubbing up and down either side of the spine as far as one can reach, producing 'friction' chi. Chi flows more easily near heat. In Summer chi flows more readily through the channels nearer to the surface of the body and in winter the chi is slower and deeper. If the pain is severe, the area can be massaged by a third party, with an active rubbing balm or enlivening essential oils of rosemary, pine, thyme, lavender, and or tiger balm. There is also 'Da Dit Jow' which is a herb massaging oil, of which there are several varieties available from good quality Chinese herbalists. This oil like the essential oils increases blood and energy circulation and is targeted at martial and sports injuries as well.

To alleviate muscle, tendon or joint pain and damage, always massage in the direction of the flow of chi, as prescribed in Massage 2) above. To bring down a swelling, rub in a circular yin anticlockwise action, whereas a yang clockwise action will enliven, this can be along a muscle or around a joint. For back pain, massage with a preferred choice of oil along the course of the urinary bladder meridian (*fig.9*), and any sore areas with the idea of activating the chi back along the channel or the painful spot in a yin or yang fashion, depending on the desired result. The above herbs, oils as well as sea salt and seaweed, can be used in baths morning and night to assist circulation.

Exercise and Chi Kung

Bladder and Kidney chi flow through their respective meridians from 3.00 p.m. to 5.00 p.m. and 5.00p.m to 7.00p.m. (GMT UK or local solar time). So, practicing Chi Kung, Tai Chi or any gentle exercise between these times is beneficial for the chi and the internal organs. By contrast the organs and their chi is on the ebb between 3.00 a.m. and 7.00 a.m. but it is still very rewarding to practice at these times. However the morning chi is yang and more protective, building anti-pathogenic energy, reinforcing the immune system naturally, as well.

Exercise gently in the manner of Tai Chi Chuan, Chi Kung, Yoga, 'gentle' walking in nature or pleasant natural surroundings and swimming in clean chemical free water. If possible try to exercise or take plenty of good quality fresh air especially morning and early evening.

Exercise should always have the motive of rotating the joints in a large gentle circle, for example whenever possible do as many of the following. Firstly roll the ankles, then the wrists, rotate the knees, elbows, hips, shoulders, neck and head, in this order from bottom to top.

Always try to keep to a dry environment and avoid stressful situations, whenever possible as these deplete internal energy. Experiment sparingly with saunas or steam baths to help dry out the body, besides yangising the body and the kidneys, they will assist the detoxifying process. This should be done by gentle trial and error, also adjusting and balancing liquid intake carefully so as not to undo the yangising process by drinking more liquid than one expels. Also being careful not to lose too much fluid too quickly or over compensate one's thirst by drinking excessively. Although saunas may reduce the symptoms of osteoarthritis temporarily, one should gauge their frequency carefully as it could give rise to more discomfort by over contracting the joints.

The following recommended Chi Kungs will depend on the level of discomfort and the length of time of the complaint. Even if one is in pain one can carry out these Chi Kungs seated or lying to great effect, from Part 3 being :- 1), 1a), 2) & 3). Then as one progresses, one can advance to 6), 7) & 8). The Chi Kungs are more dynamic when carried out standing, but both methods will be very helpful. If there are muscular problems in the lower limbs, the standing method is more beneficial and if possible done on grass, because this activates and improves the lower energy centres in the legs and feet, connecting directly with the energy of the earth.

Summary

Muscle and joint problems are engendered by excesses of yin and yang, due to the aforementioned reasons such as diet, sport's injuries, stress and so forth; therefore one must first centre the body's energy with a balanced yin yang diet (*See* Yin Yang Diet). Take regular gentle exercise. There is a Chinese saying that a hinge will not rust if the door is used. A centred diet will allow the kidney and liver to work naturally, thus the internal energy that feeds the joints and body tissue will return to a balanced state. Therefore the joints, their cartilage and the synovial fluid will be returned to a more natural condition. Extreme yang foods and substances over yangise the kidneys and their energy function, preventing them from carrying out their magnificent job of filtration and osmotic balancing. In Complementary Medicine, the kidney function is responsible for all the energy of the body as well as being the protector of the skeletal structure. So when working properly, one feels good and healthy. Excess yin substances inhibit liver function, preventing this miracle organ from detoxifying the blood amongst it sixty or so other chemical functions as well as being the protector of the muscles, tendons, sinews and interstitial tissue.

When the body starts to return to a more balanced condition, do not suddenly revert to 'old' ways, as the body will always be susceptible to the same weaknesses. But one must not live a life of denial so a balance must be struck. Therefore if one understands and adheres to the principles of yin and yang, it is far easier to balance food and lifestyle whether at home or abroad. Also to alleviate lower back trouble, one can energise and free the area by gently rubbing up and down either side of the spine as far as one can reach, producing 'friction' chi. (*See* the Bridge exercise in the section on back and neck pain).

Whenever time and occasion permit enjoy natural surroundings in clean fresh air in a pleasant stress free environment, as this alone will assist these amazing organs to maintain general heath also offering a longer, better quality of life without dependency.

Always check with a medical practitioner if you are going to take herbal remedies whilst taking prescribed medicines.

Menopause

Symptoms and Causes

Menopause is the final cessation of menstruation and therefore the end of a woman's reproductive cycle, but certainly not her individual creativity. This change is a biological statement, informing a woman to focus her life on herself, instead of the possibility of childbirth. Therefore as a rebirth, it allows women to give birth to their own inner being, after devotion to a family or a career. The popular term "change of life" is tarred with the incorrect stigma of a physical, mental, and sexual deterioration. Whereas it is new life for the woman, a beginning, springing from the consummation with her inner potential. Dr. Jung always considered this change to be a natural rite of passage into the true acceptance of the animus or male soul of a female, but in a more conscious fashion. Thus being an initiation to the numinous aspects of life.

The menopause usually occurs between the ages of 45 and 55 years, when the life force that feeds the ovaries, wanes after about thirty fives years of hard work. This change is brought on by a progressive decline in ovarian function due to the changes in the reversal of the expansive energy or chi levels of the woman. This is a natural process as life progresses, so designed in order that a woman may refocus her intentions. When these expansive, yin, chi levels diminish, the energy it takes to produce the ova decline as well. Just as day turns into night.

This natural event can have a social stigma, derived from the modern human weakness of not accepting the metamorphosis from the material to spiritual values.

However medically, menopause is an end of the female reproductive cycle. During the reproductive years, follicles in the ovaries mature and release their ova periodically by hormonal control from the brain. In the years immediately preceding the menopause, firstly some of the follicles and later all the follicles fail to rupture and release their ova, as the expansive internal energy wanes, controlled by the hypothalamus and the pituitary gland. The failure to ovulate results in a disturbed menstrual pattern. A woman may miss a period or two and even suspect pregnancy. The continued decline in ovarian activity may provoke prolonged intervals between periods or irregular bleeding episodes. The length of the periods can vary, and the flow may become either more scant or profuse, depending if the woman is too yin or yang.

Yin-Yang and The Lunar Cycle of Menstruation

A normal balanced pattern of menstruation is twenty-eight days, allied to the lunar cycle. If a woman has menstruation in a cycle, less than twenty-eight days, she is a more yang type. Whereas when the menstrual cycle is greater than twenty-eight days, the female organism has become more yin, the longer the gap, the greater the yinnisation. The same rule applies at any age. At the onset of menopause, the internal energy of an older woman has become more yin normally, causing the time between menstruation to also increase naturally. At the other extreme, female athletes or intense career women, have a shortened menstrual cycle, sometimes disappearing completely, due to the increased activity, here the female organism is more yang, causing the female hormones to become yangised or emasculated, by the overly yang or strenuous activity.

Equally, if a woman's period is greater than four days, she tends to be more yin than a female who has menstruation that lasts less than four days. A more yang woman will have her periods between the new moon and full moon, whereas a more yin woman will menstruate when the moon is waning between the full and new moon. Therefore irregular menstruation is caused by extremes of yin and yang in the diet and lifestyle, such as stress factors. Please remember yin and yang are relative. Therefore a woman who has a long period with excessive bleeding, during the waning moon is more yin, than a female who has a short menstrual cycle with a brief, light menstruation during the waxing moon and so forth. When the internal energy is altered, for whatever reason, making it more yin or yang, it will have a corresponding effect on hormonal activity.

During this change the ovaries decline in function, producing smaller and smaller amounts of the hormone oestrogen, due to this natural process of yinnisation during later life. This decline in oestrogen initiates subtle rearrangements in the hormonal activity of the glands that control the reproductive function. The decrease in output of oestrogen also disturbs the neurovascular mechanism of the hypothalamus and probably initiates the vasomotor changes that may provoke some of the characteristic "hot flushes" of the menopause. However the flushes are mainly caused by errant internal energy. The residual effect of the generative chi that was targeted at the reproductive organs and breasts, now rises upward away from its habitual zones. The chi still adheres to the vessel of conception/Renmo (*fig.14* CV.1 - CV.24), but now this excess energy splays outward, giving rise to the hot flushes. Rearrangements in the hormonal activity of the adrenal and thyroid glands also take place, for the metabolic activities of all these glands are interrelated. In most women these adjustments are usually made without too many physical or mental disturbances.

Hot Flushes and Chi

The errant chi causes a sense of warmth over the upper chest (*fig.14.* CV.17), which can spread to the neck and face and may extend over the entire body, sometimes giving rise to a prickling or itching sensation. It can cause a sort of involuntary blushing, which is usually disturbing, if not understood. These flushes can happen frequently during the night and may interfere with sleep. It can engender insomnia because of a chilly sensation and perspiring. These are all the result of the internal energy flowing up and around the 'conception vessel' which connects the reproductive system, the breasts and the mouth up the front line of the body.

Proof of the effect of this errant energy along the Conception Vessel, is demonstrated by the younger woman has had her ovaries removed, giving rise to an 'early' menopause, which is artificially induced by the surgery and not by declining hormonal function.

The hot flushes and most of the pre and post menopausal symptoms can be greatly relieved and controlled by specific Chi Kungs and diet. (*See below*).

A variety of other symptoms can and do occur, although many can appear unrelated to the changes incidental to the menopause. Nervousness, headaches, and dizziness are common complaints. The fear of ageing, the altered pattern of life, loss of sexual drive and changing family relationships also may precipitate many disturbing symptoms. Many women complain of weight gain during the menopause usually engendered by using food as a complementary comfort. Occasionally this is related to decreased thyroid function, due to poor diet and lack of exercise. Osteoporosis is a common complaint during menopause, being unnecessary, as it is caused by an unbalanced diet prior to and after the menopause. The yin yang diet will improve this condition plus the specific remedies given below.

Menstruation besides being the vehicle for discharging the unwanted ova and its by products is also an excellent way, that nature provides for a woman to dispel toxins. This is generally why a woman can be moody or suffer headaches before a period due to the change in energy, thus disrupting hormonal activity. This naturally creates emotions because of the loss, of a part of her very being, burdened by the additional discharge of toxins. When this additional cleansing mechanism ends due to the menopause, women have to ensure that the vital organs are kept healthy in order that the organism can cope with the extra work.

Cure and Diet

Therefore the vital organs of the lungs, bowels, kidney and liver need to be kept in tiptop condition, especially during and after a dramatic change, like the menopause. The kidneys and the adrenal glands which are a major hormone factory of the body, are stimulated by the hypothalamus and the pituitary gland. The adrenals also create a supplemental oestrogen, acting as a necessary back up, being able to replace the loss of oestrogen production by the diminishing capability of the ovaries. So care of this magical area is vital for life and well being. (*See* Chi Kung Section). In Complementary Medicine the kidneys and the adrenal glands not only produce many beneficial hormones needed during the change of life, they also control the stability of the bones, and if their internal energy is balanced it will prevent osteoporosis. Their function is impaired by salt, animal protein, dairy foods, and acidic fruits and foods, yang chemicals such as food additives found in meats like sodium nitrite etc. and drugs, and excess liquid above ½ - 1 litre.

The liver has over sixty biological functions being mainly responsible for clearing the blood of toxins. The internal energy of the liver and gallbladder is also responsible for vision, control of headaches etc., muscles and tendons and is adversely effected by all sugars, confection, chocolate, yin chemicals like agri-cides, drugs, and alcohol etc..

The lung and the large intestine are paired in Complementary Medicine and need to be conditioned by sensible cardio-vascular exercise in clean fresh air coupled with a balanced diet, including the necessary roughage, (*See below*).

These vital organs work together, therefore if one or any are impaired, the system becomes overloaded creating many of the known symptoms of the menopause which can be avoided.

The yin yang diet should be strictly adhered to avoiding animal protein whenever possible, until any or all the symptoms subside. More digestible protein sources should include fresh fish and organic 'GMO free' soya products like tofu, soya milk, organic soya sauces which should replace salt as a seasoning,

Therefore the dietary emphasis should be centred around a whole grain diet, preferably organic brown rice, tofu (bean curd made from soya), lentils, fresh fish, fresh vegetables including the calcium rich turnip greens, kale, broccoli, mung beans, sesame and sunflower seeds or by products including the unrefined oils made from these seeds. Also there is the Greek sesame seed paste called tahini which contains much more digestible calcium than milk or cheese, it can be used as a spread or in cooking as a thickening or flavouring. Always try to avoid processed foods and chemical liquids like diet drinks, regular tea and coffee and complicated alcohol. Avoid exotic fruit and vegetables including oranges, bananas, tomatoes, spinach, potatoes, aubergine and eggplant, rhubarb and undue amounts of citrus fruits, as these will encourage many symptoms by their yin, negative effects on the hormonal function.

The herbs that can help replace the reduced oestrogen, are ginseng with Royal Gelée, Agnus Castus, clivers (goosegrass) and Lady's Mantle. Ginko Biloba and rutin will boost circulation, easing the hot flushes. Natural diuretics like nettle will also supply useful mineral contents including calcium and iron, as well as other the natural detoxifiers, like broom, sage, bladderwort, burdock, fennel and dandelion which can be drunk as herbal infusions, acting as mild diuretics. Valerian and St. John's Wort can be imbibed to help calm the system. An overworked thyroid gland can be eased by taking kelp tablets, thus easing the hot sweats. Evening primrose oil capsules thins blood reducing blood pressure therefore can ease hot flushes, black cohosh eases menopausal and menstrual pain (contains salicylic acid thus a 'natural' aspirin effect, red clover acts as an antispasmodic and anti-inflammatory herb, all of these can help with the symptoms of hot flushes. N.B. Try one at a time and always check with medical practitioner if you are going to take herbal remedies whilst taking prescribed medicines.

Exercise

The Chinese proverb that the hinges of a door, that are well used, will not rust, is an excellent philosophy in order to maintain homeostasis during any physiological change. Therefore regular light exercise in the form of walking, swimming, gentle aerobics, leisure tennis, bowls and cycling and so forth can only help. Tai Chi Chuan and Chi Kung are also excellent exercises because they are not only weight bearing movements which maintain bone mass, but specifically stimulate the flow of the internal energy and thus ensuring a smooth transition of the hormone function during menopause. Some of the most healthy clusters, comprising millions of elderly persons, are to be found in Okinawa and a province of Fukien in Southern China. Here they eat grain based vegan diets including organic soya by products as well as practicing Chi Kung and Tai Chi. These women do not experience any negative menopausal conditions at all.

Tai Chi and Chi Kung besides being efficient cardio-vascular forms of exercise, focus on specific acupoints by way of their intrinsic movements and posture, ensuring such areas as the hypothalamus and the pituitary gland, the kidneys being the organs and glands that control hormone production, as well as positively stimulating the liver and lungs.

There are several Chi Kungs from Part 3 which will alleviate many of the menopausal symptoms. Firstly Chi Kung 1), 1a) & 1b) will control the errant chi of the 'hot flushes' from along the Conception Vessel. These can be done seated, lying or standing preferably in the fresh air, also these can be done discretely, before the hot flush is under control, seated or standing at work or travelling etc..

The more advanced Chi Kungs 2), 3), 4), 6), 7) & 8) should only be done when feeling well, whereas 1), 1a) & 1b) can be done even when feeling run down or agitated. Nevertheless Chi Kungs 2), 3), 4), 6), 7) & 8) will have a definite rejuvenating effect as well as stabilising and strengthening bone mass when performed standing.

Massage with soothing essential oils around the abdomen and along the Conception Vessel will not only add comfort but assist the flow of energy to return to a natural rhythm.

In the morning on arising gently tap the lower back with the closed fists (back), near the Mingmen gate (*fig.14* - GV.4) and lightly tap the cranium at the Bahui point (front) (*fig.14* - GV.22). This will stimulate the internal energy, chi, to naturally produce essential hormones.

Conclusion

Hormone Replacement Therapy was heralded as a wonder cure and in the short term it can prevent many of the menopausal symptoms, but now there is a rethink amongst the medical profession as there is a link to cancer. If you follow these principles one can avoid HRT or wean oneself off it. This form of self-control will not only lead to a more secure maturity with health intact, but will also give life a new meaning without fear or dependence. This can also be a time of great creativity where a woman can give birth to her soul thus allowing her wholeness to materialise, giving her life true meaning, as well as maintaining healthy sexual rhythm if desired.

Always check with a medical practitioner if you are going to take herbal remedies whilst taking prescribed medicines.

Migraines and Headaches

General Symptoms and Causes

The word headache sums up the pain experienced in the head, by its very nature of being an ache in the head, including migraine, although clinically diagnosed differently. Migraine is derived from the old English, 'megrim' in turn stemming from Latin and Greek medical terms, 'hemicrania', meaning pain in half - (hemi), the head - (crania).

All headaches are a disruption of the flow of internal energy, the excess of or lack of which, give rise to the pain. Persistent painful headaches can in extremis be caused by tumours. This, although rare, needs assessment therefore, if pain is continuous and or in one place coupled with loss of balance, vision, or any other sensual deprivation and epilepsy, a medical diagnosis is advisable in order to have a scan.

Most 'Western' medicine discounts the irregularities of chi, relying on the snap shot symptomatic and chemical diagnosis of a complaint. Thus overlooking the fundamental or intermediate cause, being energy imbalance. Hence migraine and headaches are treated with chemicals which have an instant result, but are counter productive in the long run as they waste or disrupt the internal energy flow, thus creating a vicious circle. Long term use of aspirin, which dilates or yinnises the circulatory system can damage the stomach and disrupt liver function. Whereas the analgesics, beta blockers, seratonin antagonists and other drugs can damage liver and kidney function. Seratonin replacements can give rise to scar tissue in the heart and lung.

In Complementary Medicine, when the energy or chi, coursing to and from the head is out of balance, the result is the discomfort of a mild headache due to stress or diet, right up to the alarming pain caused by the intracranial pressure due to the rare chance of a tumour or possibly meningitis which is usually accompanied by neck ache, disturbed vision, or high blood pressure (*See* Heart Section), or the unlikely possibility of a haemorrhage due to a trauma. Although all of these can be helped by Complementary Medicine, any persistent headaches may need urgent medical attention, maybe a CT scan, in order to rule out any of these rare extremes. Therefore a doctor should be consulted, even though these are the exception. Here I shall be dealing with the more domestic discomfort of head pain which is easy to be rid of, with a little effort.

Excess of Yin or Yang Chi and Head Pain

Generally if the pain is dull and spread over the whole of the head, it usually has a yin energy cause (*See* Part 3), however if the pain is sharp, it will ordinarily have a yang energy cause. This does depend whether the constitution of the person is more yin or yang (*See* Yin Yang Diet - Part 1).

Yang headache pain can be caused by too much yang foodstuffs, animal protein, dairy food, oily fish like tuna, salmon etc., salt and salty foods, tension and stress. All of which tighten the organism including the muscular contraction in the neck and head, giving rise to tight sharp pain.

In the case of migraine, where one side of the head is hurting with various levels of visual

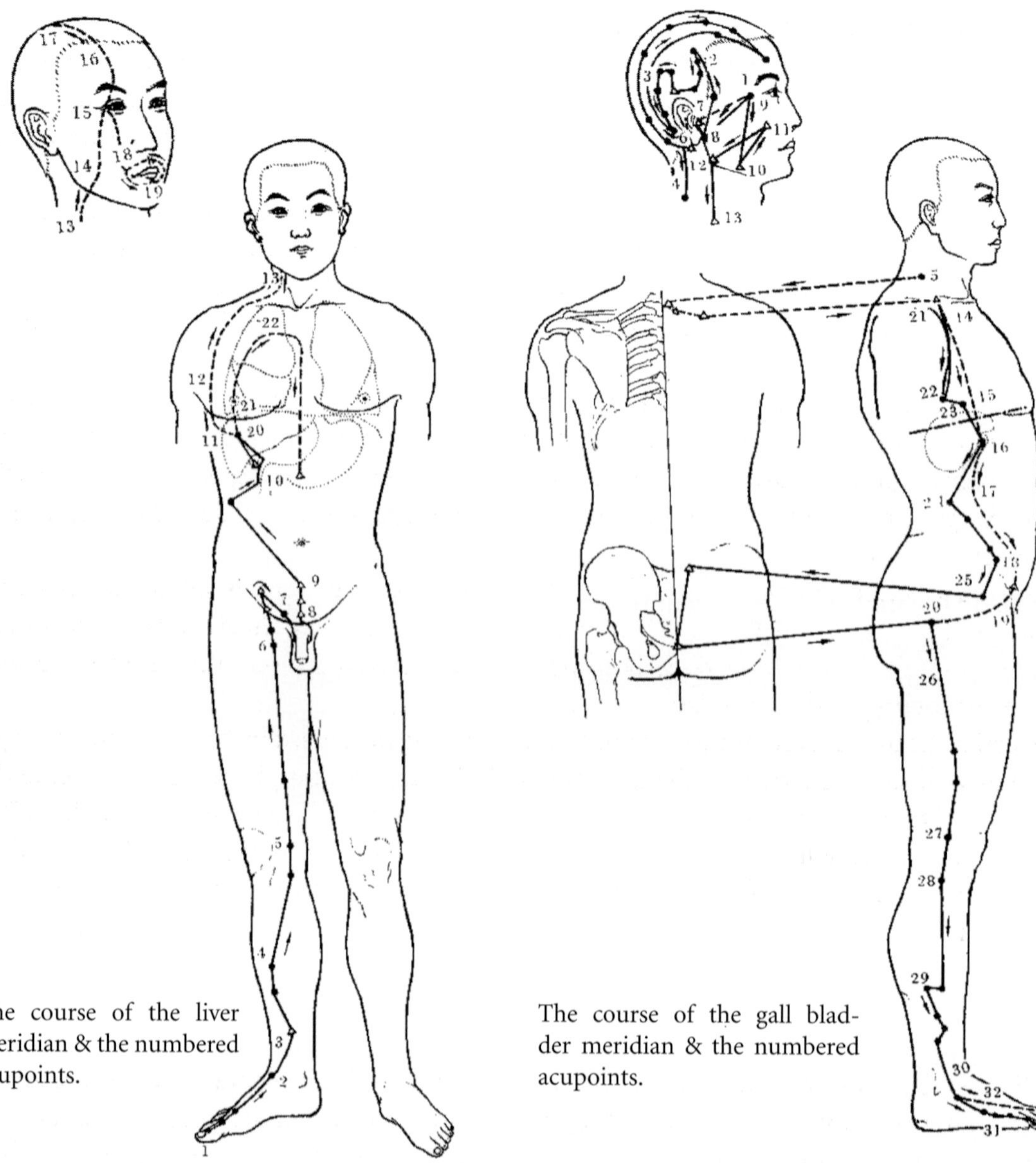

The course of the liver meridian & the numbered acupoints.

The course of the gall bladder meridian & the numbered acupoints.

Figure 10: Even if you stimulate the various points suggested with positive remedial results, if the actual liver or gall bladder are still under pressure from an unbalanced diet or stress, the symptoms will return. For yin headaches that are more dull and wide, the lower points on the foot and leg are more beneficial whereas sharp acute head pain, being yang can be more readily eased by the acupoints around the eyes, temples and neck.

discomfort, the liver and gallbladder are in distress. The gall bladder meridian has a dual circuit bifurcating along each side of the head, hence the one sided discomfort. The liver has connecting vessels up and around the eyes. Therefore if the pain is along the course of these channels, these organs are under stress disrupting the energy flow thus causing the pain, (*fig.10*). Foods that burden liver and gall bladder function are the extreme yin substances and foods, including sugar, confection especially chocolate, alcohol, drugs, food additives and colouring, spices, tropical fruit, foods containing oxalic acid (*See* Yin Yang Diet) and fatty foods as well as those with high cholesterol content including prawns and eggs.

The residual effect of liver and gallbladder stress, can be immediate as in the case of a hangover caused by too much alcohol. There are types of migraines which can be triggered by anger, depression and stress being due to the more gradual attack of these organs over a period of years by a general yinnisation of these organs. For example yin type vegetarians, especially women who have very yin diets will be more prone to migraines. Exacerbated in the female during menstruation as the liver and gall bladder step up their function during the discharge of toxins and blood. This puts an added burden on these vital organs therefore reducing the smooth flow of chi through their meridians. A balanced diet and Chi Kung will not only cure the migraines but also regulate menstruation to a normal rhythm (*See* Menopause Section).

On the other hand the more dull pains are usually a disruption of the flow of energy in the Dumo channel (*fig.14*) which runs up the spine to the head which can also be completely cured through diet, massage and exercise (*See* Cure below). This type of pain is usually caused by poor diet, bad posture, lack of or the wrong type of exercise, depression and stress (*See* Stress Section).

Obviously there can be a mix and match of both types and causes which can be cured naturally. Just as in all illnesses, an absence or excess of yin or yang chi gives rise to the physical alarm of pain. This is a warning, needing to be redressed to prevent further more serious damage occurring to the organism.

Exertion headaches are more common in men and again caused by contraction or yangisation as well as the burden on the liver and gall bladder. In Complementary Medicine the muscles and tendons are conditioned by the internal energy of the liver and gall bladder. The chi of these organs will be drained by excessive exercise, restricting the normal energy flow along the Liver and Gall Bladder meridians. This conjoined with stress, pollution, rich foods, alcohol and the modern lifestyle create ideal conditions for these types of head pain.

Cure

Ideally one should start with a detox, (*See* Detox Section). Then generally avoid excesses of yin and yang type foods (*See* Part 1), keeping to an organic grain diet and vegetables with limited amounts of animal and dairy food protein. Because dietary and emotional habits run in families there can be a hereditary disposition for migraines, so it can take an act of will to change these habits easily, but if achieved very rewarding.

If the pain is along the Liver and Gall Bladder meridians (*fig.9*), the cause is usually too much yin intake. Therefore one has to generally avoid the more yin type of foods and substances, including, sugar and confection like chocolate, as well as alcohol, tropical and citrus fruits, including bananas, yin vegetables like spinach, tomatoes, beetroot, avocados, eggplant, potatoes, asparagus, most tropical vegetables, food colouring and additives, frozen foods, irradiated foodstuffs, excess vegetable oil or oily fish, spices, diet or popular fizzy drinks, regular coffee and tea. Ensure not to burden the Liver and GB with heavy foods like dairy produce, as well as eggs and prawns.

Try and eat more organic grain food like brown rice, millet, cous cous, barley, corn, oats, buckwheat etc., balanced by fresh organic vegetables in season, with a yang inducing tendency, being the more root and firm varieties, such as carrots, turnips, swede, brussel sprouts, onions, fennel, cabbage, cauliflower, broccoli, peas, sweetcorn, green beans etc..

The more yang headaches tighten muscles and the vascular system around the head and neck so more yin foods are required. Therefore avoid heavy animal protein especially red meat, including ham, bacon, sausages, oily and salty fish, dairy food and salty foods including snacks and crisps. Increase organic grain foods like brown rice, millet, cous cous, barley, corn, oats, buckwheat and pulses. Balanced by fresh organic vegetables in season with a more yin 'open' tendency like, greens, peas, leeks, kale, and seaweed, although a variety of seasonal vegetables from the same climate will do no harm.

Try to avoid and control stress by a careful reflection of one's personal attitude to work and relationships. Events and people can trigger headaches in some. Hereditary factors can also be a cause of migraines evolving from such factors as family diets and even complexes can be passed on from one generation to another (*See* Stress Section).

When travelling, which being yang causes contraction, drink more pure filtered liquid, preferably still water, (1-1½ litres max) a day depending on activity. Try to move around as much as possible during the journey to assist circulation. This will help the body's natural system of discharging toxins and balancing energy flow. These guide lines will also prevent Deep Vein Thrombosis. Avoid rich, heavy foods like cakes, cream, ice cream, sugary confection and alcohol, even though it may give a temporary relief, because it will only make the situation worse by putting undue pressure on the liver. Keeping to a simple organic grain based vegan diet will not only prevent this type of headache whilst travelling, but will reduce travel sickness which is also connected to the liver and GB.

Herbs that ease headaches are chamomile, valerian, skullcap, wild thyme and betony, St. John's Wort, vervain and peppermint. If taken before the onset of the pain, herbs can diffuse the problem, before it fully engages. Agnus castus and evening primrose oil can relieve migraine pain during menstruation. If the pain is more dull due to vascular tightness, natural diuretics like burdock, dandelion and nettle can ease the pressure, thus thwarting the discomfort. Ginseng is excellent at alleviating 'hangover' throbbing type headaches, but as it a very yang herb it should only be taken if one's organism is over dilated or too yin.

Exercise and Massage

Whereas diet will ease the organic symptoms, Chi Kung and massage can help with the energy causation. When one feels the onset of an attack one should find a clean quiet, darkened environment and do the reverse breathing, Chi Kung 1) whilst seated or lying, then finish with 1a) as laid out in Part 3. This will help centre any errant energy and ease the energy flow in the meridians, speeding up the recovery time.

If you can find someone to massage from the yintang (*fig.14* - GV.24.5) back along the Governing Vessel over the head (GV.22) towards the nape of the neck, thus re-balancing the energy flow in this meridian. Using the first or second fingers gently massage in a yin anti-clockwise fashion on GB acupoints 1, 3, 4, 5, 6, 8, 9, 12, 17, 31 & 32 (*fig.10*). One or more of these points will be tender due to energy imbalance, a gentle massage of these points will help correct the flow of energy, thus alleviating the symptoms. Essential oils like peppermint, lavender, rosemary and tiger balm can be used in the massaging process.

The Governing Vessel can be stimulated by massaging up along the spine from the GV.4 - GV.15 (*fig.14*) helping to balance the chi flow up to the head. This can be carried out in one stroke and also by pressing gently with the second and third finger in the hollows either side of the spine, between each vertebrae.

To alleviate the more yin, "spread out" type headaches, pinch the skin around the shoulders and neck with the thumb and side of the second finger. Also gently pluck the hair away from the scalp with the fingers as well as pinching the scalp itself. This will help correct the chi flow through the head channels, which will ease the pressure of the pain.

Conclusion

Prevention is better than cure, therefore remove stress from one's life (*See* Stress Section) and deal with depression as suggested in the Chronic Fatigue Syndrome section earlier. Ensure that one maintains a balanced diet of good quality fresh foods, free from extremes along the guideline of the yin yang diet from Part 1. These precautions will not only prevent migraines and headaches but improve health and lifestyle all round. Regular exercise that is not strenuous will keep the physique and organs in good condition. Tai Chi, Chi Kung and Yoga are more calm methods to achieve this aim, but any exercise, preferably in fresh clean air, that does not put undue strain on the body will be beneficial.

Always check with a medical practitioner if you are going to take herbal remedies whilst taking prescribed medicines.

Skin Trouble - Acne, Psoriasis, Eczema and Athletes Foot

The skin is the largest organ of the body that holds the whole organism together, so one way or another if the skin is dis'eased', this vital body seal is damaged allowing pathogens and discomfort to prevail or enter the system. Skin can be adversely affected by a disturbed psyche, diet, pollution, unhealthy environments, chemical agents in soaps and shampoos, washing detergents and conditioners etc., UV light and pollution. In Complementary Medicine the lung and large intestine and their internal energy or chi control the quality of the skin and body hair. Therefore the quality of the skin will depend on the quality of food and air as well as the capabilities of the aerobic and digestive functions.

The skin acts as the barrier between the inner sphere of the body and the outer physical world. This elastic sheath holds the inner biological structure of organs, blood vessels, muscles and bones in place without which, one would literally fall to pieces. The skin is constantly renewing itself to accommodate growth, injury, changes of temperature and so forth, thus displaying any disorder relatively quickly. The top layer of skin, the epidermis consists of living cells and dead tissue sometimes referred to as the 'horny layer. Most house dust is the residue of this process, being dead skin. The skin also acts as a device to help maintain body temperature reacting to the cold (yin) by becoming yang and contracting and to heat (yang) by yin expansion and sweating. The colour of a suntan is the aftermath of dead skin, which in this case is used as a protective measure, where the skin pigment melanin being yin, is activated thus darkening the skin as a counter measure to the rays of the sun which are yang.

Skin Deep

When the skin is diseased, there is often a personal trauma at the bottom of it. Skin complaints like psoriasis and rashes often appear directly after a stressful encounter. This can be explained in the following manner. Psoriasis is a condition where there is a rapid turnover of cells in the epidermis, up to seven times more than normal which is usually about three to four weeks. This rapid cell production, instead of being discarded inconspicuously, is deposited as the scaly residues being the all too familiar symptoms of psoriasis.

Skin, at whatever level, is constantly being renewed by a person's DNA, which is recognised by Complementary Medicine as being engendered by the chi or internal energy (*See* Part 3). Chi is linked to the psyche so when a problem occurs in the psyche or soul, which is too uncomfortable to tolerate, it can manifest itself as a mutation or disturbance. This interferes with the normal replication of the DNA responsible for skin cell reproduction, aided and abetted by other additional factors like gender, diet, pollution and environment etc..

Please bear in mind that every person is different, so these disturbances manifest themselves differently depending on the person, race, environment, diet and so forth.

An extreme example of this type of disruption to the surface of the skin is the case of the stigmata. This condition occurs when the body bleeds, for no apparent reason in the accepted areas where the hands and feet of Christ were nailed to the cross. This is a classic example of a psychological form of telekinesis, effecting the body by auto-hypnosis. This is caused by a sympathetic reaction in the devout follower, by enacting a symbolic 'Imitatio

Christi' of the suffering of the incarnated God. This act of dedication causes the psyche to engender the DNA to replicate in such a manner that the skin and blood act out this inner devotion. This apparently mysterious ability of the psyche which is not consciously accepted, probably accounts for many so called miracles. Although there will be certain happenings that will always remain a mystery, like the Universe, itself. The Tai Chi masters developed their intrinsic health and martial systems by exploiting this ability of the psyche to intermingle with matter.

Skin From The Deep

Thus in psoriasis, when the skin erupts, there is a repressed disruption in the psyche, breaking down the protective barrier between the inner region of the anatomy and the outer world exacerbated by diet and lifestyle.

This shedding of the outer shell is to be found in fairy tales, which always carry a concealed meaning or lesson. Myths and legends from all over the world tell of trolls, wood spirits, mermaids or animals that can cast off their skin or tails etc. in order to change or become human and so forth. In nature the snake is constantly changing its skin to survive and throughout history, it has always been associated with evil, the underworld and the unconscious.

So when the unconscious or dark possession is truly accepted and realized, a skin dis'ease' like psoriasis will disappear as quickly as it came. If an immediate soul search and conscious making process are not possible, being the norm, dreams will direct you to the core of the problem. (*See* Stress Section).

All disease is a sickness of the soul, one way or another. People usually need all sorts of medical assistance and support to arrive at a cure. But Dr. Jung sums up the meaning of life when he wrote, 'the body is the mere visibility of the soul and the soul is the psychological experience of the body'.

Therefore never take a mishap as negative, but rather as a learning curve, this way life retains its true purpose, for without tension there is no growth. Thus turning a negative happening into a positive event.

Another example of unconscious harm to the skin, is when one cuts oneself. If one reflects at the circumstances around the time of the incident involving the sharp object, one will be able to trace a thought or an event that happened simultaneously. Possibly a sharp thought gave rise, to a psychic blind spot, distracting one's normal caution or skill.

Acne Vulgaris

This is the medical term for acne, being an inflammatory disease of the sebaceous glands and hair follicles characterized by comedones (blackheads and whiteheads), papules, pustules, nodules, and pus-filled cysts on or under the skin on the face, neck, chest, or upper back. Thus uncomfortable complaint is generally considered by mainstream medicine to be an over secretion of sebum. Predisposing factors include mainly diet, cosmetics, stress, steroids and other drugs, mechanical skin irritants like harsh soaps and washing powders and conditioners, and of course climate. Acne usually begins in puberty and affects about eighty percent of adolescents in some form. Males are affected more often, but when occurring in females it is more severe and prolonged. I have noticed that spots will occur on salient meridians and acupoints, probably because there is a lack of internal energy around that point which will cause the eruption. For example if too much liquid or alcohol is drunk spots will often appear along the course of the urinary bladder meridian, (*fig.10*).

The superficial causes are an increased activity of oil production and the size of the sebaceous glands which causes 'Intrafollicular hyperkeratosis', and the hair follicles in the sebaceous gland are blocked as comedones consisting of sebum, keratin, and microorganisms are formed. As these comedones enlarge, they become visible and palpable on the skin's surface, often forming cysts. The enlarged follicle eventually ruptures and the contents are released into the dermis, setting up an inflammatory reaction and forming abscesses.

The symptoms of superficial acne include comedones and pustules. Deep acne is characterised by inflamed nodules, pus-filled cysts, abscesses which if prolonged can cause minor scarring of skin tissue.

Spots, Diet and Lifestyle

The main cause of acne in Complementary Medicine, which has a high success rate in clearing acne, without the use of drugs, is to modify the diet. Acne is caused by too many toxins, remaining in the blood being excreted by way of the pores of the skin. This happens because the usual routes are impaired, being by way of the liver, kidneys and large intestine, which are the body's main source of discharge especially in the male. Acne is prevalent during times of hormonal activity due to the increased biological drain on the internal energy. As every person is unique, different foods will effect people in different ways. The main causes in the diet will be due to over consumption of some or all of the following, excess liquid especially alcohol and 'soft' drinks, fatty foods, dairy food, 'junk food-burgers, fried chicken etc.', too much animal protein, excess amounts of sugar from sweets and sugar by-products such as jams, industrialised foods including battery eggs, chicken, pork, beef and vegetables and fruit, grown with high levels of chemicals including pesticides and fertilisers. Stress is another factor that can spark off acne. Stress will burden the kidney energy thus reducing its function to clear out toxins, (*See* Detox Section).

Unfortunately the over-stressed medical services tend to prescribe drugs being a quick fix and for acne usually prescribing tetracycline anti-biotics, called minocycline, the trade name being Minocin, and to a lesser degree bactericidal creams and washes. This will sometimes have an effect, but as drugs have to be taken out of the system by way of the kidneys, this type of treatment can do more harm than good in the long run. Creating an unnecessary burden on the internal organs, thus producing a vicious circle. It has now been accepted by the medical profession that anti-biotics can reduce the immune function.

Simply follow the 'Complementary Medicine diet' detailed in Part 1, try and reduce stress, and avoid chemical substances in the diet and in all washing. Eat foods from natural sources grown or reared without chemicals, pesticides, hormones, artificial colouring and preservatives. i.e. avoid 'junk foods' and keep to a diet of about - 60% of foods comprising of organic whole cereal grains. Grain foods such as brown rice and buckwheat are good for the digestion and circulation, plus all the whole grain foods, to add variety, are acceptable. Only eat natural whole wheat bread whenever possible. This can include limited amounts of naturally produced organic, animal protein, including free-range chicken, duck, non-oily fish and sea-

The 5 Phases of Change

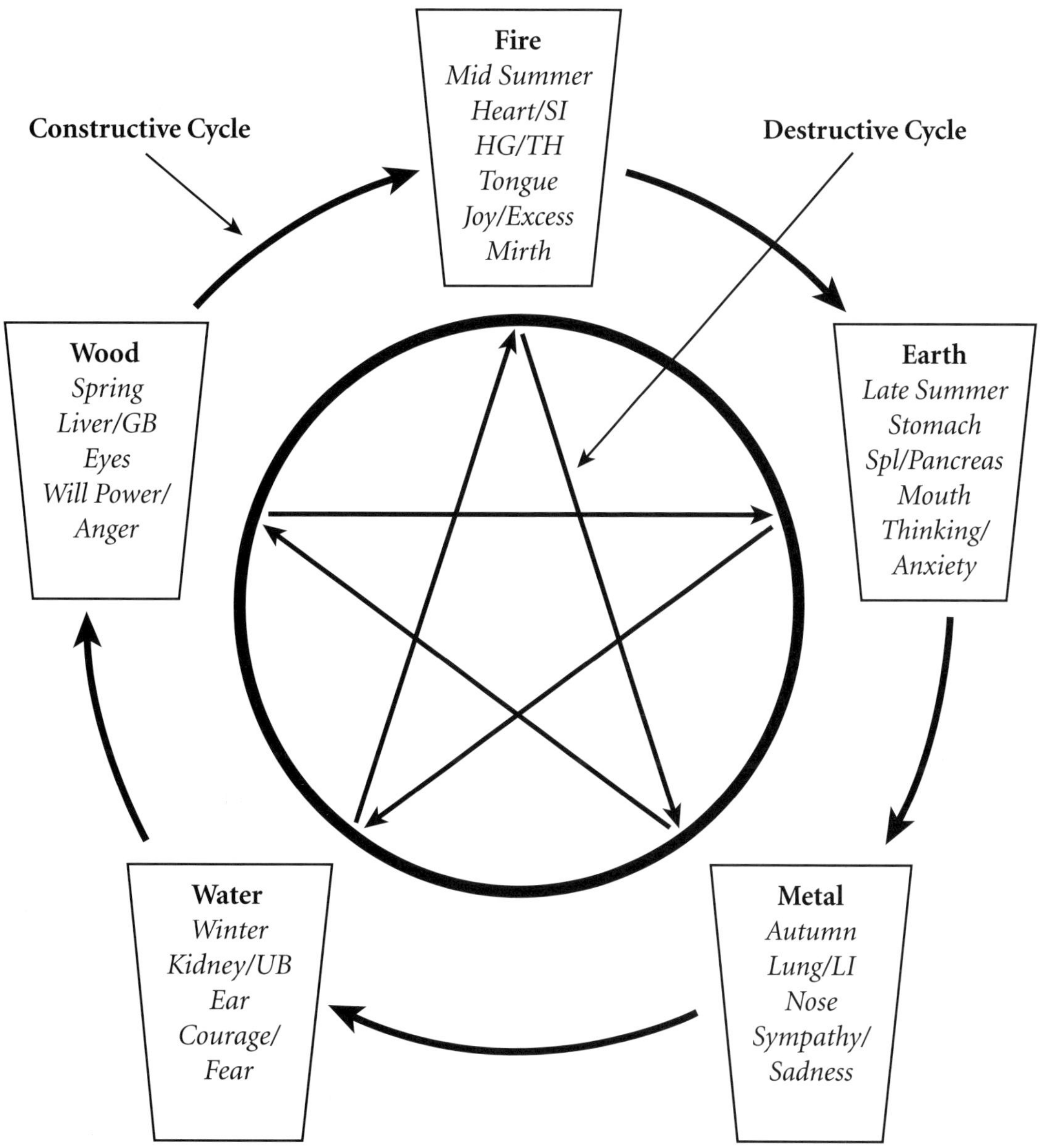

Figure 11: The Five Phases of Change albeit laid out c. 5000 years ago in The Yellow Emperor still has a relevance today in diagnosing and observing the human condition.

For example, the energy potential of the summer is related to the internal energy of the heart and the small intestine organs, in such a way that during the summer these organs are recharged. This phenomenon also applies in the micro-cosmic daily cycle of midday. The day being a microcosm or fractal part of the year etc.. Even in today's more conscious world, the emotions are connected to the internal organs, i.e. if the kidney energy is weakened by diet or stress, one is more fearful, having a tendency to tremble or shiver in the manner of water. Also the internal organs can be affected by the related negative emotion, so if one is made very sad by an outer event, it will deplete lung energy etc..

Often one can find that the energy of an internal organ is depleted by a host of related phenomena, connected to the relevant time of day, season and emotional upset, because the inner and outer are inter-related in a synchronistic way. this is due to the fact that the psyche and matter are linked at all levels including our well being, because the body is the mere visibility of the soul and the soul is the psychological experience of the body.

food (no prawns). Red meat is to be avoided as it is very difficult to digest, clogging up the digestive system and thus slowing down the elimination of toxins. The yang aspect of the diet should include a balance of plant protein in the form of about 10% of pulses including split peas, chick peas, beans etc.. The 20% yin of the diet must include fresh organic vegetables especially greens, including broccoli, spring greens, leeks, salad greens, cauliflower, green beans, carrots, celery, turnips, swede, organic salads + 5% indigenous fruit in season, excluding citrus fruit, (except lemons occasionally *See below*). The last 5% of the yin balance should be a liquid intake of ½-1 litre a day depending on activity, in the form of pure uncomplicated fluids including, filtered water, herb teas, like burdock and dandelion.

N.B. Avoid all dairy foods (cheese, milk, butter and eggs), spices, junk food, food and confection containing sugar, especially chocolate, soft drinks, jams, and diet drinks and foodstuffs that have additives, preservatives, colouring and chemicals. Regular tea and coffee should be avoided whenever possible. Acne sufferers will notice the skin is worse, a day or so after too much liquid, especially alcohol.

Keep away from all acidic foods and citrus fruits and spices (except controlled amounts of lemon *See below*) and tropical fruits and foods and tomatoes and their by-products and spinach, eggplant, aubergine and potatoes.

Depending on taste, cook foods simply like 'stir frying' so as not to waste the nutritional benefits. For recipes, buy vegetarian cook books but keep to the above balance of yang to yin foods because some vegetarian diets are far too yin and contain exotic or tropical taboo foods.

Herbs that are helpful adjuncts to clear acne (*See* Detox Section) include rosemary, thyme, chervil, celery, tarragon, chive, fennel, cumin, capers, nutmeg, clove, horseradish, wild thyme (serpolet), saffron, dandelion, parsley, sage, burdock, bladderwort, and nettle. Pokeroot is also a tried and tested herb for the skin.

Wash the affected areas in tea tree oil, in preference to the powerful chemical bacterial products generally available on the market, as although they will kill the bacteria, long-term use will be harmful to the skin. Also avoid harsh personal washing powders (biological) and body soaps, preferably use pH balanced products for personal hygiene as well the pH balanced non-perfumed washing powders and fabric conditioners. Always wear natural fibres, particularly next to the skin.

Echinacea, which boosts the immune system, can be taken carefully, but if after two weeks there has been no improvement, discontinue and try a mix and match of the other herbs, either as infusions or with food. The juice of one fresh organic lemon in hot water and honey each morning will help, but must be used only in warm weather, otherwise one will over yinnise the organism.

Acne is far less prevalent in hot climates where food is more natural and traditionally prepared.

Try and take plenty of exercise which is not over strenuous preferably in clean fresh air. Many toxins are absorbed into the system from the polluted environments in the towns and the cities. Whenever possible allow the effected areas of the skin to be exposed to the air. When on holiday, skin problems heal more readily due to stress reduction, the body being more exposed to the elements and also one tends to wear less clothing etc.. Sea bathing is excellent for toning the skin and ensuring its healthy renewal. Always use a good quality natural sun tan lotion as some contain many chemicals, being harmful. Look out for the 'parabens' additives as there is research in the US to show these are carcinogenic. Saunas and steam baths will help detox the skin and the body's toxins.

Psoriasis

This is ignorantly declared by the medical profession as being incurable, because the psyche is not taken into account as well as diet and environment. I pointed out earlier in this section, that all disease is a sickness of the soul one way or the other. With, 'the body being the mere visibility of the soul and the soul being the psychological experience of the body'. Therefore, in Complementary Medicine, to ensure a cure one must be rid of the underlying reason buried in the psyche. (*See* Stress Section).

In Complementary Medicine the energy of the skin is controlled by the 'Five Element' visceral chi of Metal of the lung and large intestine, supported by the Water internal energy kidney and urinary bladder. To keep homeostasis of the organism if only one part is treated, the cure is limited, because there is a dual circuit of energy in the body that can be disrupted. Firstly the internal energy flow of the twelve main meridians, attached to the vital organs, should be worked on, on a daily basis and secondly by way of the 'Wu Hsing; (*fig.11*), where the chi of the internal organs is interdependent on various cycles, including the seasons.

This diagnosis is born out, albeit unconsciously, in Western medicine by the following facts. Often there is a streptococcal infection, a sore throat, before the onslaught of psoriasis. Stress is also given as a cause and psoriasis is often accompanied by asthma, in severe cases there is psoriatic arthritis. In Complementary Medicine the kidney energy controls the immune function and disorders of the skeletal structure, whereas asthma is caused by poor lung chi.

Therefore, in order to relieve the symptoms in tandem with the soul search, one must balance the internal energy especially of the aforementioned organs. The balanced yin yang diet must be adhered to, with an emphasis on clearing the bowel by reducing yeasted breads and increasing organic whole grains to be about 60% of the diet, especially organic brown rice, barley, oats, millet, corn and cous cous. Brown rice which contains phytin acid is an excellent detoxifier, (*See* Detox Section).

Animal protein and dairy food must be avoided, as they clog up the digestive and respiratory systems. Junk food is particularly bad for skin trouble due to the reduced nutrition and high chemical, fat, oil and sugar content used to bulk out and flavour the poor quality food. These interfere with kidney function. Keep away from industrialised foods containing preservatives and chemical additives. 5% of the yang element should be comprised of protein from pulses, as found in chick peas, lentil, bean and GM free soya beans etc.. This will ensure a balance of natural protein input which is assimilated easily by the body. The amount should vary according to metabolic rate, more activity, more pulses and so forth.

Skin Food

Healthy skin thrives on good circulation and blood which needs plenty of fresh seasonal organic greens including cabbage, cauliflower, broccoli, brussel sprouts, green beans, kale, seaweed, salad greens and a balance of organic root vegetables. This should be about 30% of the dietary intake.

The last 5% of yin substances should include fresh organic fruit, in season, excluding citrus fruit, including a sensible amount of clean uncomplicated fluids, about 1/2-1 litre a day, depending on fluid loss (sweating) and activity. Too much fruit and fluid will slow down kidney and bowel efficiency.

Taboos, Herbs and Skin Bathing

Avoid the taboo yin foods including citrus fruits, tomatoes, potatoes, rhubarb, spinach, spices, eggplant, aubergines, strong alcohol, sugar and its by-products, all soft drinks with chemicals and or high acidity and sugar confection and by products. All of these make the blood acidic which will reduce the body's ability to produce healthy skin.

Herbs that help cleanse the system are burdock, bladderwort, dandelion, nettle, rosemary, milkthistle, thyme, mint, meadowsweet, elderflower and chamomile. Nervines including, skullcap, valerian and St. John's Wort will ease stress, helping to fortify kidney chi. Echinacea can be tried out for a month at a time to see if this eases the condition.

Dead Sea salt baths stimulate and soothe the epidermis, as do 'pure' bathing products containing, aloe vera, evening primrose, comfrey, jojoba and tea tree oil. Saunas and steam baths can help detox the system and aid healthy skin cell renewal by increasing circulation.

Plenty of fresh air and exposing the skin to the elements will drastically improve the symptoms, (*See* last paragraph of the Acne Section), but exercise must be specific and not strenuous as this will deplete kidney chi. Tai Chi and the following Chi Kungs will fortify the internal energy and strengthen the immune function as well as the chi of the bowels, kidney and lung, from Part 3 :- 1), 2), 3), 4), 6), 7) & 8). One should try and do a mix and match of these early morning and evening when the chi of the intestines and kidneys are flowing respectively, including the Tai Chi, which being a moving Chi Kung will reinforce the structure of the skin and the keep the joints in good condition (*See* Joint Section).

Eczema

This has two causes one is external from chemicals and is also known as contact dermatitis, usually more prevalent in persons with a lower protective resistance due to the reasons cited in the psoriasis section, exacerbated by stress, poor diet, hereditary factors and pollution. The effected areas can be cleansed in products containing aloe vera, evening primrose, jojoba and especially tea tree oil. External application of chickweed and chickweed ointment will assist the healing of the skin tissue. If the reason is not a chemical irritation, then it is caused by stress and poor diet. Applying the same remedies as for psoriasis will cure the complaint by removing the toxins from the blood which are being discharged onto the skin as the kidney, liver, lung and bowel are burdened. (*See* Detox and Stress Sections). The diet and Chi Kungs applicable for curing psoriasis will cure eczema. Eczema is also triggered by harsh washing products for clothes, baths foam, soaps and preparations. One has to buy and use natural products from specialist stores. The regular simple soaps and so called 'dermatologicaly' tested products are useless.

A University Professor of Dermatology was nagged by his young son to buy a supermarket child's bubble bath which was packaged in order to attract children. He bought the child's product and when home swapped the contents for a natural product. As he did not wish to waste the child's bubble bath from the supermarket he washed the dog in it. The dog then contracted eczema. I also wonder what was in the dog's dinner.

Athlete's Foot

Known medically as tinea pedis, describing the fungal infection of the toes and feet. The reason why some people are more likely to catch the infection is because the immune function is under par. This is due to poor diet and stress which reduce the immune function. The yin yang diet should be adhered to especially trying to reduce junk foods, animal protein and dairy food. These foods are also the cause of smelly feet which usually accompany athlete's foot. This is caused by stagnated blood and reduced kidney chi responsible for anti-pathogenic chi which is yang and protects the surface of the skin. Athlete's foot is more common amongst those who wear trainers because they creates a local unnatural, yin environment aided by sweaty feet, allowing the bacteria to take hold and multiply more readily.

Despite a change in diet and careful hygiene and the wearing of cotton socks, in order to reduce the symptoms and prevent cross infection, one can apply topical herbal remedies of tea tree oil, aloe vera, thuja and witch hazel that will help clear the fungal infection effectively and naturally. Echinacea will strengthen the immune function thus attacking the infection from within. Depending on diet and effort this should take no more than a month to clear.

Always check with a medical practitioner if you are going to take herbal remedies whilst taking prescribed medicines.

Stress

The hustle and bustle of life not only distorts the true meaning of our existence, but the very words we use to go about our daily business. Stress, is a new age curse but if we take a little trouble to look at the actual word and its derivation, one can see a hidden agenda in its meaning and why it has been adopted to describe this present condition. It seems that mankind has only replaced the past ills for new ones.

Here I am using the word stress to encompass all the pressures that the psyche encounters in the modern world which can include the strain of work, a bereavement, relationships, depression, insecurity of personal or world affairs and so forth.

The Original Meaning of Stress

Stress was first used in the middle of the 16th Century in England being derived from 'distress' which in turn comes from the French word 'destresse' via 'distrain' from the Latin 'districtus' meaning divided in mind. There are many other offshoots including, 'straits' as in Straits of Dover, describing a narrow or restricted stretch of water, or the phrase 'goods in distress'. A legal term from the past, still used in law today, when goods are seized or distrained to offset a debt, thus causing distress. Stress can also describe the pressure on a human being or an inanimate structure such as metal which will buckle when over stressed and so forth, but always denoting a strong onslaught of focused tension.

Today, more than ever the medical profession accepts that stress is detrimental to health. It is responsible for a variety of problems including; reducing the ability of the immune function to operate efficiently, encouraging colds and more severe illnesses as well as physical trauma including cancer, bad backs, weak muscles and tendons, organ dysfunction, especially heart and lung trouble, IBS, stomach disorders, allergies, skin complaints etc.. Stress also impairs the mind to operate appropriately. These two areas of physical and mental stress are now prevalent everywhere.

However some types of stress can be positive, in manageable doses, being a necessary teacher which can fortify and stimulate development, because tension produces growth. This necessary tension has been and still is a character builder of mankind and a selective evolutionary tool in the natural world. However too much stress is a danger because the intensity becomes overbearing and destructive inwardly to an individual's mind and body or expressed outwardly as collective disasters and war.

That Which Does Not Kill You, Makes You Stronger

A classic example of this potential, explosive tension was expressed in the work of Frederich Nietzsche, the German philosopher, whose writings were a source of disastrous inspiration for the German Nazi movement in WWII. He pointed out; "that which does not kill you makes you stronger". Unfortunately all too literally for Nietzsche as fate took him to an early grave, jilted and torn apart by a broken heart, afflicted with venereal disease. He became split or stressed by his genius which he thought was his own. Whereas it came from the unconscious.

When stress becomes too much for a person, it becomes destructive, however disguised whether on a personal plane or in society as a whole. This syndrome can lead to selfish hedonism which covers up the fear, provoking a form of self deception, in order to justify the 'I'm all right Jack' attitude, all too prevalent today. In short, individualism which is one of the mainstays for global injustice and environmental destruction. This short sighted view not only blindly ignores the plight of the less fortunate, but above all, maintains a disparaging blind spot towards nature. These synthetic and superficial forms of compensation can only end in disaster for the individual and society. There is a golden rule that if one tucks away an uncomfortable truth in the dark recesses of the psyche, it can only manifest itself in a negative manner in the world of light. This rule applies to both the individual or the collective. Thus we meet our darkness as fate in a disastrous manner, whether as personal or collective crisis.

There is a simple solution that will not only relieve the individual but help the collective as well. If one takes a fresh look at the whole situation, the solution for this divisive stress is to be found at the core of the predicament. Let us return to the original meaning of the word to 'narrow' or further back 'divided in mind'. One can see that the root meaning of the word, is a split. This division fractures the ability of the person to handle dilemmas in a balanced fashion. Surprisingly with the best will in the world, positive thinking will and can never work because it is one sided. For, if the negative is not accepted and realised, this dark element will control the situation in the end, by way of projection. The unconscious always projects through the individual, until reflected or caught with the mind by honest self-analysis. Therefore all this modern stress is really a manifestation of the individual or collective strife engendered out of unconscious projections.

Stress will never be relieved by modern science, even though it can mechanically highlight relative areas of the brain, with the aid of 'scanners' which pinpoint centres of activity caused by stressful events. However the CAT scan does not explain the emotional differences between people and how each person reacts differently to life and its problems.

Brain, Tool or Centre?

A scan can identify the electrical activity of the all-important, hypothalamus as well. A region of the forebrain, which amongst many of its functions, stimulates the anterior pituitary gland to produce adrenocorticotrophic hormone, ACTH. This hormone, in turn triggers the production of adrenaline, the main 'stress' hormone. But this science does not show why one person will be scared and produce adrenaline for one reason, yet another person will have no reaction.

Also there are the medical stimuli, including drugs, which turn off or subdue certain areas of the brain's activity, but this technology does not address the difficulties of life, character and so forth. The medication merely numbing the brain as an expedient method of subduing the symptoms. These immediate quick fixes do not address the whole person, often leaving the patient with disagreeable, long-term side effects.

It is obvious that stress effects people in many differing ways, some people thriving on it, in a sort of masochistic fashion. Whereas some are split apart, whichever the case, both are detrimental in the long run. The question is where does one look for the answer? Doctors, therapists and the media are full of any number of superficial solutions including, exercise, meditation, diet, holidays, alcohol, drugs, counselling, change of lifestyle and so forth, all having varying different levels of superficial success.

The method I will lay out is suitable for any person who is willing to take a bit of trouble in examining themselves. This will not only resolve the conflict, but also give true meaning to life itself, because the solution always lies at the heart of the problem. The problem is how to access this centre. Initially this can be awkward because although the dilemma holds the key, it is hidden behind a blind spot. Even though this blind spot can be very evident to enemies who can exploit this weakness. On the other hand, the well meaning, but the all too often unwanted advice of family and friends is often ignored. However the key to unlocking this mystery is available to all, completely free every night, in dreams. Because dreams are personal, they can be more poignant than any other stimulus. (*See* ***Time for A Change***).

Jung and Stress

The first person to uncover this dream factor, in an empirical way, was the Swiss analytical psychologist, Professor Carl Gustav Jung (1875-1961). He discovered this remedy, conclusively at the beginning of this century, after his exhaustive studies of the mind, the psyche, dreams, history, religion, philosophy, mythology, folklore, Western and Eastern alchemy.

Historically, Jung has often been wrongly associated with the Freudian school of thought. Although Sigmund Freud was an early mentor for Dr Jung, he soon parted Freud's circle because the young Swiss doctor found Freud too rigid in his view of the psyche and dream interpretation. Jung realised that Freud, although a pioneer in the field of psychoanalysis, could not address the deeper, mysterious realms of the human being, where religion and science meet. Also the psyche's ability to 'see' into the future or contact other people at great distances and so forth, plus containing the meaning of life.

Jung's research proved how buried in each psyche there is an objective autonomous core, which can guide any person, willing to look inwards. This not only heals any split, but also gives a true meaning to human existence. He determined that there was a totally independent and personal arbiter in the dark areas of the psyche. He called this area of the psyche, the unconscious because one is not aware of its contents. He proved that dreams are the method of communication between the two worlds. Because dreams are expressing unconscious contents, their language has to be symbolic. This language of symbols is necessary in order to bypass the blind spot, expressing allegories from religion, poetry, ancient myths, folklore and fairytales. Thus dreams point to the missing 'half' of a person, acting as a balancing and compensating arena.

Stress and The Unconscious

There are two main levels of the unconscious, firstly a personal unconscious and deeper down in the psyche is to be found the collective unconscious, where the archetypes dwell.

The personal unconscious is where we tuck all personal events pleasant or repressed. This area nowadays is fairly easily aired with a little self-honesty, by education and open discussions with a partner and friends. It also contains archaic remnants of survival techniques which evolved in order that our primitive ancestors could perpetuate their species, before collective societies. This explains the selfish gene syndrome. Unfortunately these methods

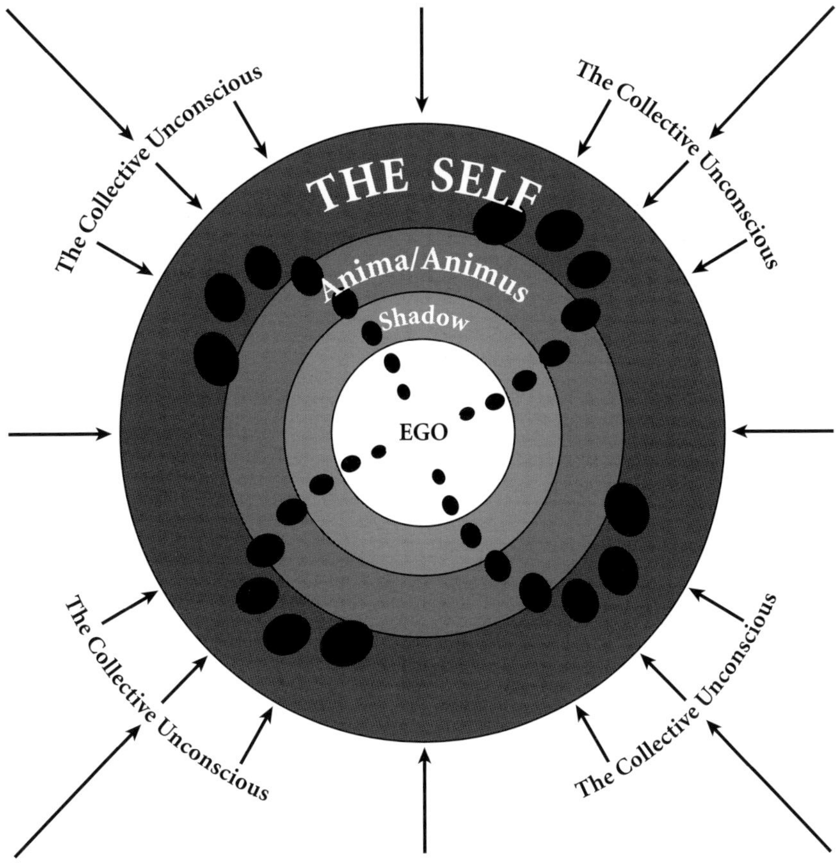

Figure 12: **Schema of an Introverted Psyche** - It is impossible to depict the indescribable, but Fig. 20 is such an attempt. In this diagram the ego is placed at the centre because it is figuratively at the centre of consciousness, being a complex of experiences formed at around the age of seven, when a child differentiates himself or herself from parental influences. This is when 'we' becomes 'I'. The ego continues to expand during life at different rates depending on the ability of the person to differentiate opposites. Consciousness is not about intelligence, but concerns the ability of individuals to acknowledge opposites from the personal and collective unconscious, including the archetypes of the shadow, anima, animus and the Self.

The first layer Jung called the shadow, which contains character traits that are unacceptable to the ego, hence repressed. The saint has a sinner shadow, whereas the criminal has a policeman in his shadow. However, when shadow characteristics are accepted truly into consciousness, the ego becomes stronger and the old shadow traits will be useful 'friends' acting as an excellent form of self defense. In dreams the shadow will usually appear as a threatening character of the same sex, often depicting a person one dislikes.

The anima and the animus are the contra-sexual aspects of the psyche, which act as guides into and out of the unconscious. These parts of the psyche are the stuff love is often made up of. The anima of a man is often projected onto a female that epitomises this area of his psyche and vice versa. When the anima and the animus are distorted, deviations occur such as impossible love matches like Romeo and Juliette etc. or homosexuality. The animus of a woman is conditioned in early childhood by a father imago, whereas the anima is fashioned by the image of a mother figure. When acknowledged these archetypes guide one into a meaningful existence and the absolute truth of the Self. The Self is the God Image of an omniscient, omnipresent force that is and has been projected collectively, onto Deities of both genders since time immemorial, however each person has this personal Imago Dei within. It is masculine for the male and feminine for the female. The Self will appear in dreams, in different guises depending on the level of consciousness, being a benevolent authority figure, imparting wisdom, being of the same sex as the ego. All unconscious contents are projected and have a negative effect until made conscious by reflection, through the discerning capabilities of the ego. The sum total of the archetypes originating from the collective unconscious represents individuation, i.e. not divisible, thus creating wholeness, giving life its meaning and true purpose for each individual.

of survival have developed, misguidedly, into the new dilemmas of the desire for power, opportunism, materiality, greed, selfishness, jealousy and so forth. However these initial instincts were necessary to protect food, family and the tribe against the hazards of nature and rival aggressors. But now these instincts are more or less redundant, as mankind is more conscious and able to provide and protect itself in cohesive societies. But due to levels of unconsciousness still prevalent today, there are vestiges of these prehistoric instincts that display themselves today, spilling out as environmental destruction, exploitation of people and war etc..

What goes around comes around, because extremes are linked at their weakest point. It is for this reason that religion and social codes have always dictated certain rules, not only in fear of wrathful deities, but pure common sense, because by the law of opposites, the exploiters will become the exploited. Life highlights the negative results of the projected aspect of the unconscious because one will bump into them in the cycles of fate, in the trials and tribulations of existence. This is another dimension to the universal law of opposite and antagonistic tendencies of all things; also manifesting as the old Chinese code of yin and yang.

Dark Forces

Unfortunately these old codes have to be updated, as mankind needs a new understanding of the psyche. This requires more individual consciousness, and far less collective values. I hasten to add that the 'new' material mantra of individualism, cannot work, as it is a distortion of becoming an individual. The advocates of individualism, being the powers that be, are manipulating the weaker and darker side of human nature. This manipulative control of the ruling elites, by way of the biased media, is a classic case of divide and conquer. Media was first exploited in this way as a very successful marketing and PR tool, by a nephew of Sigmund Freud called Edouard Bernays in the US at the beginning of the twentieth century. This selfish side to human nature which everybody has, is exploited as a method of control. The shadow is manipulated by big business and politicians of all hues especially nowadays by the new credo of the worship of the market force and the debtor society. This demonic condition and all its dire effects, is in effect a collective shadow situation. It is this aspect of the personality that is easily manipulated by the controlled propaganda of politicians and the media. This divides society into selfish fractured entities by inducing fear in order to maintain the order of power. This is the tried and tested theme of divide and conquer. However because this principle is based purely on egotistic values, which contain projected shadow criteria, it can only end negatively.

Consciousness and Enlightenment

One can, only truly, form into an individual, by developing more consciousness. This can be achieved whilst still supporting the collective, by being a responsible and decent member of society. Unfortunately, nowadays, shadow qualities are encouraged and rewarded by increased material gain. This attitude perilously ignores our fellow humans and the environment. The results of which are all too evident, and what happens when the shadow of the one and a half billion Chinese et al, is let loose on the world?

The personal unconscious is really an instinctual, upper echelon of the collective unconscious. The psyche is formed out of an archetypal structure, which is made up of four main areas. The first is the ego complex which is the centre of consciousness (*fig.12*). It is like an island floating above a vast ocean. The meaning of the word complex has been distorted by psychology and its very relationship to this area of the psyche. It actually means, a coming together (com = *cum.* Lt.) of many things (*plex*), be it expressing the ego or a repressed set of circumstances. i.e. like the collection of factors that create an inferiority or mother complex. Complexes manifest themselves as irritable moods, tantrums, depression and uncontrolled tempers, obsessive behaviour, etc..

The ego is a fusion or complex of features and experiences formed into a cohesive entity, at around the age of seven years. This usually occurs when a child starts to identify him or herself as a person. Quite often children say 'we', prior to this, as they identify themselves with the egos of their parents, family or social group.

The human ego complex is the reason that homus erectus contains a unique level of consciousness which is different from all other species. Therefore the Darwinian perspective of the ascent of man should really be replaced by the evolution of consciousness as opposed to the survival of the fittest by natural selection. Intelligence and education do not create or guarantee consciousness, on their own, although they are necessary. It is wrongly assumed that a high intellect is a higher form of consciousness. Consciousness is actually a fusion of opposites, formed from the understanding and marriage of these conflicting tendencies. The unconscious is a chaos of undifferentiated opposites, seeking the light and actual manifestation through the discernment of the ego complex. The ego has the ability to marry these inner and outer conflicting halves, if not, they are projected. There are many, so called brilliant academics who do not appreciate the all too evident opposites in nature or in the psyche. Remember the atom bomb did not grow on a tree, it came from the psyche and thus the unconscious.

The Ego

This ego, being a complex of opposites, is derived from the collection of experiences, gathered together throughout life. It is born out of parental influences, racial and religious origins, environment and childhood occurrences. All this information is fused together by the inner being, the soul, of an individual. As the person grows, the ego enlarges its field of consciousness by absorbing conscious and unconscious experiences. Therefore consciousness is relative to the ability of the ego to consciously assimilate the split halves from the two spheres of the psyche.

The Shadow

The next layer is the shadow, so called because it is something dark that lies in the shadow of the ego, just under the threshold of consciousness. This negative side of the personality, always has a destructive tendency, when left unconscious. This is because one always projects unconscious contents out into the world of people and matter, until one reflects on these subjects in the magic mirror of the mind, thus making them conscious. This is why we meet out unconscious as fate.

In reality, individual or collective conflicts are the effects of unconscious projections battling themselves out in the material world.

A simple, yet uncomfortable way to identify one's own shadow qualities is to look out for a person of the same sex or similar personality who has all the qualities one dislikes. This may be housed in one or several persons mirroring our own repressed and rejected traits. For example a very manipulative person who is constantly weaving selfish plans in the shadows, will clash or will accuse others of being control freaks. Often such people are petrified of snakes, spiders and creepy crawlies as they represent their own clandestine qualities. The shadow can appear in dreams in these forms. However with a little honesty, if such a shadow trait is accepted, it can become a positive aspect of the psyche and create a consciousness with great organisational abilities. The shadow is only hostile when ignored or misunderstood. For example a bully who has a cowardly shadow can become brave, the person with feelings of inferiority can become heroic, an idler can turn his or her life around by positive activity and so forth. The personal or collective values of the unconscious are a compensation for the attitude of the ego, so whatever is on top is a compensation for what is underneath. The shadow is therefore just a distortion of survival instincts that have become the all too recognisable failings of humanity now played out as duplicity, stealing, violence, jealousy, power drives, greed, selfishness, hubris, sexual deviation and so forth. The shadow appears in dreams as the same sex as the dreamer and is often at the core of nightmares appearing as dark and menacing characters. The Christian shadow was exemplified in the New Testament as Christ's shadow The Devil. The Shadow of Mary the Virgin Mother, has a projected shadow as the fallen woman, Mary Magdalene.

The Inner Guides - Anima and Animus

Underneath the shadow one discovers the inner guide, which if left unconscious, has random and nefarious reactions in both men and women thus disturbing consciousness, unexpectedly. However, when accepted and realised is an inspiring ally. In women it manifests itself as a masculine figure and in men, it is female. The male side of the feminine psyche is called the animus whereas the male has an anima. The animus and anima are the contrasexual personifications of the respective psyches. In classic literature they appear as demons or witches in their negative or projected condition, but develop into inner guides with the possibility of divine inspiration, when made positively conscious. Jung realised that if the anima or the animus is projected it causes a host of love disasters. However when integrated into the consciousness is a guide into and out of the deeper reaches of the unconscious psyche. Writers, composers and artists depend on them for inspiration. For more humble folk, these inner navigators can help us through life's ups and downs, smoothly.

Mythical Anima

In dreams the anima will be in female form, often appearing as an ideal female partner who can inspire the male and lead him into and out of the unconscious. A good example of a legendary anima figure, is Ariadne who gives Theseus a magic thread to guide him out of the tortuous maze, where he slew the Minotaur. Here the female is a benevolent anima guiding the hero in and out of the darkness so he can conquer his negative or beastly qualities. Another classic depiction, this time a negative anima, is the Gorgon Medusa with her terrifying hair of snakes whose gaze would turn any man to stone. Perseus aided by his polished shield was able to kill her, by sighting her image in the reflective qualities of this magic screen. These simple well known legends, show in story form that if the anima is kept in the dark it will have petrifying effects, but when reflected upon is helpful, creating a hero out of the man.

In life when the female side of the male is kept in the dark or is negative the man is frozen from reality finding the big bad world only a mess that is not worth bothering with. She will keep him in dark moods, depressed, weak, spiteful, fickle, vain and above all, unattractive to real women.

The anima is conditioned by the relationship to the mother. Therefore if there was a negative experience or total lack of a mother figure, the anima will have those qualities which in later life are projected onto women who will live out the negativity, thus giving rise to bad relationships. This does not mean that this experience has to be all bad. If the anima is brought to the fore instead of lurking around in the dark areas of the psyche playing all her tricks, she will become a good creative friend. This leads to strong positive bonds with women and life. In order that a man give birth to his anima proper, it needs the accompaniment of an open minded woman, preferably someone who understands the idea of the unconscious, i.e. she accepts that she has an animus. If not the anima and animus will battle until one or the other of the partners, just buckles under the strain. This is not healthy as the so-called winner will live in a precarious hubris, whilst the other remains lifeless. In the case of the anima of a man, it is the hen pecked husband. All love quarrels are made of this stuff and have been in evidence all over the world since time immemorial. The anima is tied up with the sexual energy of the body and of course, is the true food of love.

If the mother imago has been too positive and possessive this can lead a man to having shallow relationships such as the Casanova attitude to women, where the man can never allow the woman in or have a deep contact with the female, because it is tied up within his anima. Also this type of mother complex can lead to a man having only one woman in his life, his mother. Thus his love and sexuality is bound up and projected onto men with similar complexes. This type of gay man is usually very creative and has a high feeling content and if openly accepted, it does not have to be detrimental to his development. Often in these gay unions, one man is more feminine than the other, creating a balance of sorts. Jung says the increase of homosexuality came to pass for a variety of reasons including overpopulation, as well as a collective need for men and women to embrace part of their shadow complex, i.e. loving and embracing the same sex. However, it is down to personal choice and it's effects.

The anima as well as being the inner 'inspiratrice' and cohesive substance for relationships is the inner guide to the centre of the male psyche, the God Image of the Self, which is always masculine for the man.

Animus, Legend or Legion?

The animus in a woman, if neglected can become legion. Especially in this modern age of so-called equal opportunities. The female is now more than ever dependent on her masculine soul, in order to face the trials and tribulations of modern life. If the animus overwhelms the female ego, it can cause the woman to become frigid, dogmatic, reckless, full of empty talk or silently frozen, obstinate, dangerous and so forth. These destructive animus qualities can sublimate, the very creative and now necessary aspect of the female psyche, being the feeling function. The animus, if made conscious and realised, give women a superior advantage in the new world with the added quality of retaining all the wonderful aspects of femininity. Besides making a woman naturally confident with all the organisational abilities needed nowadays, the conscious animus will compose positive ties with the opposite sex and children. Just as for men, the animus really needs a partner of the opposite sex for it to be truly recognised. This can be achieved through a close relationship, friendship or counselling.

Animus and Bluebeard

Just as the mother shapes the anima of a man, the animus of the woman is conditioned by the father, hopefully giving her a clear concise way of ordering all the aspects of her life. But the negative animus will appear as a bluebeard type character in dreams, robbing and murdering her femininity. Bluebeard was a mythical character; the stuff fairy tales are made of, based on an actual sixth century Breton chieftain who killed his many wives. In the fairy tale he is a rich prince who lures young maidens into marriage, forbidding them to open a secret door. Just as curiosity killed the cat, a new young wife cannot resist the temptation. Therein, she finds the dead bodies of Bluebeard's past wives. But here her curiosity saves her life as she uncovers the murderous aspect of her husband in time. Another classic example of the destructive animus is in Wuthering Heights, where Emile Bronte in her one and only book, projects her negative animus into Heathcliff. He torments Bronte's heroine, Cathy, in a love hate relationship which continues even after her death, showing that this character is paranormal.

Whereas the male personification of the female psyche, when enlightened, will be her best friend. This is laid out in the fairy tale of beauty and the beast. When the possessed and entrapped girl, can embrace the beast, he turns into Prince Charming, the man of her dreams, and she lives happily ever after.

Most religions being patriarchal are of little use to the modern woman or at best a stepping stone. Whereas the older nature cults have more in tune with the feminine psyche where Goddesses were worshipped and served the female, so the true way is to find the Goddess within which is a major leading role for the animus.

The Self and The Centre of The Psyche

This positive animus will open the way to the spiritual union with the higher aspect of the psyche, the Self. The Self is female for the woman.

Jung pointed out that if the world was to survive, it would be due to the feminine and the feeling function. (*See over* and *fig.13*).

The Self for both men and women is the ultimate goal of human existence. It is the Image of God and the centre of the human psyche. The Self can only, truly be realised when the shadow and the animus or anima are made conscious. However a path towards the Self can be activated by guilt which usually occurs after a trauma. A raw encounter with the Self will be recognised, never to be forgotten, as it can be awesome. A mild manifestation of the Self can be felt sometimes as a temporary feeling of well being or oneness caused by a number of 'happy' occurrences such as the warmth of a family gathering, winning a prize or an event, promotion, creative endeavours and so forth. For the Saints, it was a dramatic experience, the 'Ectstasis' or ecstasy.

Over the centuries people have sought out this elusive spirit, in many forms even misguidedly, from the 'spirit' in the bottle, with alcohol being the hidden inner spirit, and also drugs. A modern sickness is the scourge of alcohol and drug abuse in many consumer societies, with some substances even being falsely labelled 'Ecstasy'. The devastating 'worship' of materialism and all the other 'ism's' are another area which needs correcting to ensure a secure future for subsequent generations. These are all a 'loss of soul' and an unhealthy projection of the archetypes of the unconscious.

The Self and Dreams

The Self appears in dreams as the same sex as the dreamer in the guise of a positive authority figure. This varies according to the consciousness of the dreamer, it can be a teacher, doctor, monk, nun, priest or even a stereotypical version of a God or a Goddess from an accepted religion or cult. Jung pronounced that when the Self spoke it was the voice of absolute knowledge, often ignored, but it is the free will of each person to listen or not.

There is a caveat as always, because along the path of self-discovery, involving the complexes and archetypes, there is a personal price. However when identified as a natural occurrence, is less disturbing than when it first appears, for if recognised it can be controlled. This is a mild depression. When the centre of consciousness absorbs these dark elements, the light of the ego is dimmed, thus causing a slight depression. This is necessary to allow the effect, and the unconscious contents to congeal into the world of light. If this is repressed, it will only appear at a later date in another fashion, usually more destructive. Jung discovered that when life has no meaning one day and meaning the next then you know you are on the Via Regia.

It is extremely dangerous to accelerate this phenomenon by artificial means such as mind-altering substances. Although in many native cultures a ritual lowering of consciousness was controlled by an experienced medicine man. Alas many of these rituals have been lost, along with the knowledge of the shamans, leaving many native cultures to fall into depravity.

Certain Indian tribes from North America sometimes ritualised this rite of passage in their 'sweat lodges'. On occasions using mild hallucinogens to assist the transmutation from one existence to another. On the other side of the Pacific Ocean, the shamans of the Australian aborigines admit that the demise of the traditional life style and degeneration of their peoples, is mainly, due to the loss of the rituals that can contact the 'dream time'.

This altered state, is not to be confused with manic depression or a psychosis which must be treated as an illness because the ego has lost control, albeit due to an unconscious eruption. In such cases the island of consciousness has been overwhelmed by the waters of the unconscious. It was not by chance that Western Alchemy used the sobriquet of Mercury for this domain with all the allusions to lead and quicksilver. These substances were not only pseudonyms for the unconscious but its potential quality of being poisonous. The curse of the genius is that he or she is precariously close to the unconscious. This can explain their bizarre, even mad and sometimes short existences because the unconscious, although a source of inspiration can overwhelm the ego, if care is not taken.

Positive Depression

This listless feeling of mild despair, if understood, then controlled, can be exploited to improve our well being, because when the ego potential is diminished temporarily, it opens a door allowing in these illuminating features. These factors then enlarge and strengthen the ego making it more fertile. Thus the island of consciousness grows, rather like the layers of congealed lava surging up from the depths of an oceanic volcano turning from a barren landscape into a balanced and diverse eco-culture.

After a lifetime of experience adopting the Jungian method of analysing dreams and the psyche I acknowledge, as Jung determined, there are no fixed laws to elucidate the unconscious, but there are certain archetypal components which are more or less common.

Dream Sample

Here follows a 'made up', possible dream of a man, containing some basic, archetypal themes. The genders can be reversed for the feminine ego.

'A man is walking on a sea shore where he encounters a black magician who scares the dreamer, for it appears the evil wizard wishes him harm. He flees into the sea to escape, where after nearly drowning, he is rescued by an enchanting mermaid who carries him off to a sacred island. There, she introduces our refugee to a wise old man who is a white magician, living in a cave. The helpful magician whispers secrets into his ear and gives him an amulet to control the evil magus. He notices, much to his surprise, that both magicians have the same features'.

The man is our 'make believe' dreamer. The seashore is the border between the unconscious, represented by the sea, and the conscious, terra firma of dry land. The black magician is the man's dark shadow personality, which is always the same sex as the person who dreams. The shadow of an individual is easily, but painfully recognised in dreams or otherwise in life by being those characteristics which we dislike in another, usually of the same sex. The shadow, as all unconscious contents, is projected and destructive until being made conscious by reflection. People often create a false persona or public face, which acts like a mask covering the darker shadow personality, often revealed in a person's laugh.

In this example, the mermaid (half human, half fish) being the helpful anima figure acting as a positive aspect of his feminine soul. In myths and folklore the mermaid has had two aspects on the one hand, helpful, the other, the siren luring sailors and their ships to crash on to the rocks. The anima can also be devastatingly irresistible, the 'femme fatale' which destroys the man because he is chasing a dark, destructive projection of his own soul. The anima is conditioned by the mother imago, so it often occurs when a man has had a negative experience of motherhood, he is easily seduced by actual sirens or indulging in impossible liaisons, also sometimes personified in the form of the unobtainable 'She' of Rider Haggard, such as beautiful women, actresses, pop stars etc., always, much to his chagrin.

The benevolent anima can be exemplified in myth and literature as the 'inspiratrice' for a man, much as the Muses were to the Ancient Greeks. These nine daughters of Zeus and Mnemosyne (memory), encouraged the creative spirit in man to the fore, inspiring poetry, dancing, songs, painting, the art of love and so forth.

Oedipus and Electra

The Oedipus complex is now a cliché for men, where the man loves his mother incestuously, thus destroying him and her. But for women, there is also the lesser-known 'Electra complex' which is an unresolved conflict with the father, giving rise to pathological relationships with men. In Greek legend Electra was the mythical daughter of Agamemnon and Clytemnestra. She convinced her brother, Orestes to murder their mother and her lover, Aegisthus, in retaliation for the murder of her father, Agamemnon. Thus the conflict began for her and gave rise to the 'Electra complex'. This type of complex can lead to poor unions with the opposite or same sex.

The Self

The wise old man for the masculine ego in this case is the Self. The Self is only the image of God or the Creator, due to its unfathomable potential, aptly summed up by St. Augustine who described God *'As a circle which has a centre which is everywhere and a circumference which is nowhere'.*

I have not delved too much into the female psyche, in print for a variety of reasons therefore I recommend the works of Dr. Marie-Louise Von Franz for further reading on the workings of the female psyche.

When trying to interpret dreams, a simple rule of thumb is to take the meaning literally first, then look at any symbolism making it an adventure of self-discovery. Remember dreams are not there to insult you but to guide and forewarn you on your path through life.

70,000 Dreams

Dr. Marie-Louise Von Franz, who has dedicated her life to Jungian psychology, was a student and close collaborator of Jung with an exhaustive workload of dream analysis, some 70,000, and books second only to the founder himself. Quoting Von Franz from a dream seminar; "The unconscious, amongst other things, is a great jester, and from time to time it speaks right out - bang! So that as you write the dream down you explode with laughter and you know what it means. Just the other day for example, I was very ill and revolting against my illness, I dreamt that, *I was at a festival to greet old soldiers coming home from military service. And as they handed in their carpenter's tools, I saw they were terribly old. They were a hundred years old, and somebody said into my ear, "Yes, they have kept those people much too long in active service".* Now you don't have to be an analyst to understand that dream. At once I drastically reduced my workload."

Professor Jung stated that an oral communication in a dream must be accepted, verbatim. Also to help understand dream language here is a brief intermezzo into Jung's four functions which are needed by the psyche to orientate itself in consciousness. (*fig.13*).

The Four Functions

Briefly the four functions can be described as follows, sensation tells one that something exists, thinking informs what it is, feeling guides us emotionally, whether it is good or bad and

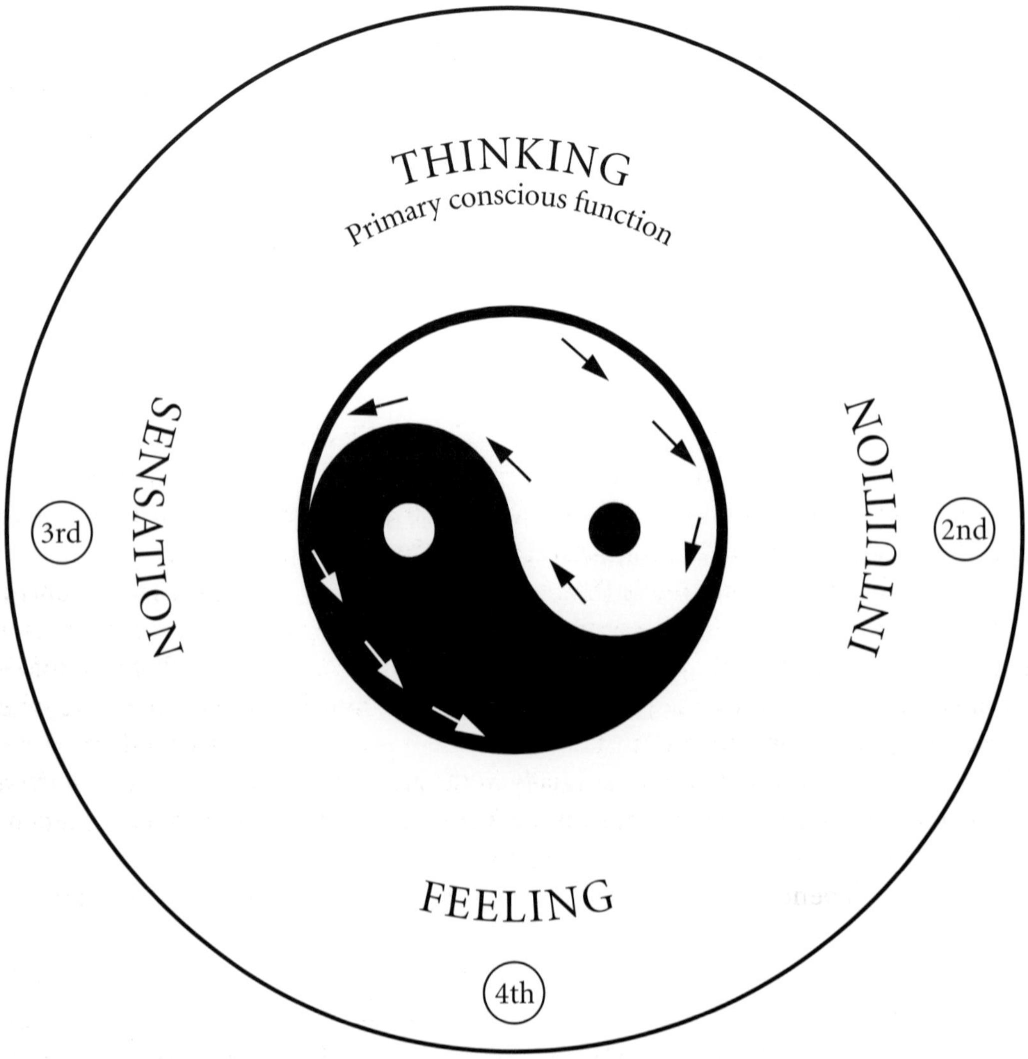

Figure 13: **A schematic diagram of a 'thinking/intuitive' psyche** - Thinking and feeling are rational functions therefore, always opposite each other. The same is the case for the other two irrational functions of intuition and sensation. The order of the functions depends on which function is primary or secondary. The order never remains static, but when one function predominates, it is the basis for 'function type' recognition. The predominance of type also adjusts with maturity and/or sometimes a trauma. Often the shadow will have traits of the secondary function, intuition in this case, whereas the lowest function will be represented by the anima or the animus which will also be the opposite in terms of introversion or extroversion, e.g. if the ego and the primary function is a thinking type who is introverted, the lower function of feeling will be extroverted attached to the anima or the animus, often displayed in an immature, outlandish manner.

intuition speculates its origin, past and future use. When intuition is accepted as a function it becomes a method of 'seeing' into the unconscious, that is 'perceiving or sensing' even the future because the unconscious is a time space void, where past, present and future are undifferentiated. Mediumistic people have intuition as their foremost function. Thinking and feeling are opposites balanced by the other two, sensation and intuition. For example if a man has a predominant thinking function, seconded by intuition, his two lower functions will be sensation with feeling at the lowest point. So the masculine ego has the two upper functions whilst the underlying ones are less conscious, and feminine allied to the anima. The anima will often appear in dreams using these lower functions.

The reverse will be true for a woman. If a woman has sensation and feeling as her lower functions, they will be her masculine attributes and attached to the animus. This type of psyche can make a successful entrepreneur or dealer.

Often people are attracted to each other at an unconscious level because the type is opposite and complimentary. Hence a 'thinking' man will be attracted to a feeling type woman and so forth.

The Fluidity of The Functions

The functions are never rigidly static, their precedence will change from time to time. This can be noticed when somebody is out of character. But, when a certain function predominates most of the time, it will fix a position for the others, determining the typology of the person. However the order of the functions can and do change during life.

Jung pointed out that thinking is the opposite function to feeling which he considered to be logical. Whereas sensation is contrary to intuition, being the illogical functions. Here illogical does not mean that they are unreasonable, but outside the norm. For example it is a well-known fact that people can dream or have accurate hunches about the future whether a businessman, dealer or a medium. If all events were purely causal it would create a dead world without inspirational criteria, especially in the arts but equally one needs a sixth sense to buy the right house. These illogical facts are just so, hence accepted logic needs redefining to incorporate this quantum field of the unconscious.

Wholeness is dependent on including all the functions into consciousness, therefore a balanced standpoint is to use all the functions equally, in a rounded way. Simplistically, take a problem, think about what it is, then use sensation to tell you what it is in material terms, thereafter intuition will determine where it came from, the past, and where it is going, into the future; lastly feeling will guide one as to whether it is good or bad thing. In this way one sees any situation or dilemma in a wholesome fashion.

Dream Ideas

Each dream is unique and personal; therefore the associations must be interpreted in this manner. However there are crossovers, so I shall lay out some general hints which are not to be taken under any circumstances, as fixed rules.

Dreams of flying indicate an inflation, one is puffed up full of air, above oneself needing to come back to an earthly reality. In a classical myth, this is clearly portrayed by the hubris of the hot headed Icarus, who disobeying the advice of his father Daedulus, flew too near to the sun causing his wax wings to melt and fall to his death. Whereas birds can point to an overuse of the thinking function whilst ignoring the opposite and balancing earthiness of feeling. Feeling could be expressed by kind, sensitive animals or people, i.e. caring mothers, nurses and domesticated animals etc.. Dogs often represent intuition as they can nose out a problem. Our canine friends can be mystical messengers, in the tradition of Anubis, the Egyptian dog or jackal god. He was also depicted as a dog-headed man attending to a 'mummy' or conducting the dead into the underworld Hall of Judgement. Here the passed over would have their hearts weighed to see if it still contained any guilt, this was overseen by Osiris. The statues of the scales of justice all over the world are derived from this mythological procedure.

We now live in a period of excessive flying both literal and figurative ignoring the feeling area of sensible compassion to our fellow humans, animals and the environment.

Water normally represents the unconscious as do forests, caves, dungeons, cellars etc. representing a sort of back door to the realm of Nature. This is evident in fairytales and myths where heroes are often lost at sea, in forests and deserts only to be helped by trolls, talking animals or weird and wonderful creatures. Being immersed in water can also mean a baptism of renewal. Drowning could indicate life's problems are too much and going over our heads.

Fire can mean a variety of things but if it is hot or burning then beware as things are getting too steamy or dangerous. Fire also cleanses and changes, bringing new life. The fire of the sun illuminates so this form of incandescence could herald more consciousness. When I first started the process of individuation, I had a dream where *'a capuchin monk, his face obscured by his cowl, beckoned me across a threshold of hot coals in a dungeon'.* A baptism by fire, which subsequently happened in the blaze of events during this process of individuation.

Earth spirits or animals, crocodiles, bulls, snakes, chthonic gods like Pan, trolls, earth dragons etc. normally relate to an unconscious instinctual side of our nature. Snakes and saurians possibly indicating a cold-blooded approach to a problem or a person, i.e. using a thinking aspect only. Bulls or Pan could demonstrate the raw sex drive of self-preservation or desire.

The Beauty and The Beast

The English patron saint and his myth, St. George and the Dragon are derived from a Christian martyr from 3rd century Palestine who was popularised by the Knight Templars on their return from the Holy Land. St. George is the hero killing off the primal shadow instincts of his power drive displayed as the dragon. This act released the damsel in distress which had been captivated by this shadow quality. This act of heroism released his anima and the Eros function of 'feeling'. This theme was acted out by many Templars who after the fruitless and bloody crusades gave up violence. This feeling function caused them to instigate the debacle of fairer legal and justice systems, charities and hospices all over Europe. Also several became troubadours wooing maidens with their love songs and poetry. Even modern Freemasonry which is derived from the Templar tradition has to have a charitable arm.

The female equivalent is the fairytale of Beauty and the Beast. Here the charming and beautiful young maiden has to embrace the beast in order to release his handsome qualities. This echoed in Sleeping Beauty, Prince Charming and the Princess and the frog.

When one dreams of a house, it can represent the psyche, the upstairs being the conscious realms and the lower floors, more towards the unconscious. Houses on fire could be danger or change. Running away is usually evading a problem. If one is being chased, the gender or type of pursuer will determine whether one is trying to escape the reality of the soul or the shadow. Death in a dream can be an end of an old relationship or facet. A pupil of Jung's dreamt that Jung had died. When he told it with trepidation to Dr Jung, he smiled and replied to the student that, now he could take on his own patients. Killing can denote a repression of an uncomfortable item; young children being a childish attitude. Whereas a birth or new born child indicates a rebirth of the individual or the birth of a complex, both paving the way for a new perspective on life. Often a dream of a child in 'my house' will represent the same age as a forgotten or repressed childhood trauma. For example if the child in the dream is three, it could be the unconscious is pointing to an incident that happened at three years of age.

Summation

To sum up, take dreams seriously, at face value, however bizarre, work on them at a sensible pace even if the significance is not immediately apparent. The soul will have registered an effect, with the meaning, possibly surfacing years later. Dreams can be treated as a drama played on our own personal stage, so the first part can introduce the theme and the characters, the next being the story line and lastly a suspended uncomfortable event. Three being an incomplete number, requires the fourth enlightening element of consciousness to unravel the meaning being the final conscious conclusion. Always write down the dreams and take the trouble to allocate associations to the contents whenever possible.

Therefore the only real combat to stress or division is to integrate the archetypes from the unconscious into consciousness and when one is contact with the Self, one's life will have true meaning and security. If knowledge is power, then self-knowledge is freedom.

Jung proved this fact time after time and only ignorance denies it. Obviously one has to be questioning about 'voices' from inside, but the 'voices' in a normal person will be the ever obliging, informative archetypes, as in the above situation. In the case of the very disturbed, being schizophrenics or psychotics, the 'voices' will be dangerous complexes which need professional analysis. Safer are the 'voices' and or their images from dreams.

Since antiquity from the Greek Tragedies or the Arab Story tellers throughout history including Shakespeare, the archetypes of the unconscious have been portrayed as the heroines, heroes and demons of literature. These acting as a catharsis, thus temporarily exorcising the unconscious projections from the psyche. This is what makes a play, opera, book, film or soap fascinating as it acts out these archetypes. For example Shakespeare's Macbeth, the word still taboo for English speaking actors. It is a story of greed, thus the shadow, motivated by a manipulative female, Lady Macbeth playing the role of the dark anima. The tale resolving itself with the hero emanating from a wood, representing the redeeming function from the unconscious.

Exercise

Any form of exercise will temporarily act as a physical ventilation for stress, however the more strenuous, the more deleterious in the long run. It is more appropriate to relieve tension by taking a break in natural surroundings, preferably doing more soothing movements like Tai Chi, Chi Kung, Yoga and less so remedial massage. These will assist the centring of the internal energies of the mind and body, allowing a welcome respite in order to create a window of inspiration to seek out the source of the problem. The mind and body need to be quiet for the unconscious to engage smoothly.

When feeling really uptight during the day or night, *Refer to* Part 3 and do Chi Kung 1), seated on a chair at work or whilst travelling or lying down. Always park the chi back at the centre, when finishing all breathing exercises with 1a) and or 1b). These Chi Kungs will not only help dissipate the symptoms of stress, but can be used to relieve jet lag as well as being an aid to sleep. Chi at night flows down from the head to the body, this is why we yawn. The yawn is expressing the exchange of energy from up to down, night to day and vice versa in the morning. When the active or yang chi is locked in the head, usually due to pressure, it causes unnatural wakefulness and anxiety. If one does the deep breathing 1) in a relaxed manner, even thinking of the feet, this will help draw errant chi away from the head. This natural energy exchange is the very core of why sleep can refresh and reset the mind and body. These techniques will realign the body's bio-rhythms which are disturbed by stress, travel, poor diet etc..

Never do any Chi Kung other than 1) and 2) until the organism is centred, then any or all of the others can be performed and will maintain health giving rise to a much more stable life.

Overview

To sum up take problems one at a time bearing in mind that they can always be resolved. Step back and away to find the epicentre of the crisis. This is like reading a weather map as opposed to being in the eye of the storm. Thus isolating the potential causes and perpetrators. Judge whether it is worth becoming embroiled in a situation in which you may only be partly involved.

Exploit the stressful situations as a learning curve, taking advantage of sensible self-adjustment, as a rite of passage from one experience to another. The centring process is assisted by balancing one's diet, exercise, environment and relationships, not forgetting the objective information which dreams can impart. Try and bear in mind that the only constant is change, attempting to remain as constant in change as possible, taking every opportunity to see the funny side of life.

One needs yang chi more in the day time for general activity and more yin energy for the night to allow healing and rest to take place. A mental exercise, which helps to release tension, is to slowly go over the problems of the day in reverse order, ticking off the various possibilities and solutions. This will prevent the mind going into 'automatic' retrieval because if a problem is let loose in the psyche, it naturally tries to seek a solution, just as yang needs yin. Therefore pre-empting this process will take away the autonomy of the anxiety.

Whatever you do, always stay as relaxed as possible and to do this one needs to 'know thyself'. Self knowledge is freedom, giving rise to more stable relationships, career, money matters and lifestyle and an overall satisfaction of life itself, not only benefiting yourself but these ripples of wholeness eddying out into the world.

Always check with a medical practitioner if you are going to take herbal remedies whilst taking prescribed medicines.

Teeth and Gum Care

The whole substance of the human body is dependent on the internal life force and its flux between its two polarities having relative states of expansion, contraction and intertwining, from soft yin to hard yang. (*See* Part 1). This law of opposites equally applies to the thirty-two teeth which are horizontal and yin, being a relative complement, to the thirty-two vertebrae of the spine, being vertical and yang. According to Complementary Medicine the teeth are composed by the yin chi of the mother and the father's yang energy is responsible for the spine. Chi predetermines DNA; this subject is covered in more detail in my book ***Tai Chi Chuan and The Code of Life.*** Basically Chinese medicine and philosophy, including Tai Chi Chuan is based on the ***I Ching, The Book of Changes,*** which sets out sixty-four major criteria. It still has valid spiritual and physical implications today, even though it was first drafted in 2600 BC.

Synchronistically, DNA has sixty-four codons, which compose the very structure of all living things. The thirty two 'yin' chi derivatives of the teeth and the yang energy that produced the thirty two vertebrae of the spine are an outer manifestation of this archetypal '64' fold structure to be found in the I Ching and the codons of DNA, matching the 64 squares on a chessboard and so forth.

Dream Teeth

Teeth can also have psychological associations because quite often in dreams if teeth are lost or damaged, this indicates a loss of control, because teeth are the front line of digestion, and thus survival. Therefore teeth have a variety of implications besides their superficial accepted function. For example their use to support a smile, or at the other emotional spectrum, the stress related grating of teeth or common phrases of chagrin like, bite the bullet and so forth.

Due to the teeth being the first part of the digestive system, the best way to care for them is to have a balanced healthy diet, on the guidelines of Part 1. Any dentist will tell you that junk food and drink will ruin teeth, even though oral hygiene of brushing and flossing after meals may be above average. It is the substances in the food and drink that cause caries, gum disease exacerbated by the dietary implications of the type of food, i.e. being yin or yang, having relative effects on the teeth and gums as well as the whole of the body.

The teeth are evolutionary indicators of how and what we should eat. The majority of human teeth are pre-molars and molars, twenty for an adult, which are best suited to grinding grains, cereals, legumes and other seeds, followed by the eight incisors advocating the eating and cutting of vegetables and lastly the four canines being the evolutionary teeth for tearing apart animal food. Therefore a rule of thumb is to have a diet which follows this ratio which works out at a ratio of five parts of grain type foods to two parts of vegetable matter and lastly one part animal protein, (5:2:1.). This basis gives rise to the balance of foods laid out in Part 1.

Here I shall explain tooth and gum care from the perspective of yin and yang. To recap from Part 1, chi is relative and is in a constant state of flux. The teeth are very yang on the outside, composed of the most yang or hardest substance of the body which is enamel. This is most effected by yin substances. The most harmful yin substances for teeth and gums are strong vinegar, all sugars, acidic food and soft drinks including citrus fruits and of course many of the chemicals used in food additives. Tooth enamel is safest when the saliva is kept slightly alkaline. This can easily be proved by the 'coke test'. Take a tooth that has fallen out and place it overnight in a glass of coke or for that matter any regular 'soft' drink, by the next day one will be able to observe that the tooth has started a process of softening and decomposition. However if the tooth had been placed in salted water, the tooth would remain completely intact. These yin inciters of decay also cause the gum to yinnise and dilate. This produces an environment where bacteria can lodge, between the gum and the tooth which can cause gum disease, as well as loosening the teeth. Teeth that decay easily are also a sign of weak bones which is caused by poor kidney energy function, which can be inherent or caused by eating excesses of yin and yang food. (*See* Part 1.).

The shape, size and formation of teeth also show how the emphasis of yin and yang can determine not only the quality, but also the way they sit in the jaw. This is dependent on the type of food eaten by the family before birth, during pregnancy and in the person afterwards.

Teeth that stick out or have gaps are a sign of a yin constitution, whereas tight small teeth indicate a yang physiology. If the teeth point in, it shows an overly yang tendency brought about by inherent consumption of excess quantities of meat or protein. Teeth that point in many directions show a chaotic diet of extremes of yin and yang food and drink over a long period, possibly initiated by the mother during pregnancy.

Toothache

There are two root causes of toothache, firstly when the gum or nerve becomes exposed due to decay or harsh and incorrect brushing of teeth. The other reason is when the nerve becomes swollen with the increased pressure inside the tooth, giving rise to the pain. Both initiated by excess yin or an expansive condition.

A simple remedy is to rinse the mouth in a solution of sea salt in pure warm water, (c. 1 tsp. of sea salt to 25cl. of water) which will clean and yangise the mouth, besides taking some ginseng which will help contract the energy of the organism, including the blood vessels, these will diminish the swelling of the gum and the nerve, relieving the pain.

The colour of the gums or gingiva being a mucous membrane denote blood quality. Healthy gums are pink whereas red gums indicate an excess intake of yin expansive foods including drugs, this will have relevant effects on the teeth.

The ideal way to maintain a healthy mouth is to eat a balanced diet, being sure to include firm foods, predominantly comprising of grains and vegetables, these are not only essential for health, but strengthen the teeth and gums, accompanied by plenty of chewing. Chinese saying, a wooden door hinge that is not used will get woodworm.

The cleaning of teeth has generally improved with the greater awareness of brushing and flossing, with an unhealthy emphasis on using chemical whiteners and bactericides in toothpaste and mouthwash. These are in effect counter productive in the long run. Modern living and diet have produced these harsh substances to counter the residues like plaque formed by the industrialised foods. Thus the harsh chemical toothpastes and mouthwashes which have a negative yin effect, eventually weaken the teeth and the gums. Also there will be a residual

intake of chemicals which are absorbed into the system by way of the mouth, thus adding to the potential cocktail of harmful chemicals, putting undue toxic pressure on the body.

Clean Diet, Clean Teeth

The best way to keep teeth clean and the mouth alkaline is to brush with finely ground sea salt or occasional use of denshe. Denshe is Japanese for a tooth powder made out of an equal amount of finely ground roasted sea salt and carbonised aubergine, preferably prepared in a mortar and pestle, as electric grinders can yinnisc the mix. As the paste is black it can yellow the teeth if used daily over a long period. Although it is very effective at cleaning and yangising the teeth and gums, it does not whiten teeth.

Sea salt especially, or any natural yang medium will not only ensure an alkaline presence in the mouth, but also act as a very effective bactericide. Also it tightens, by virtue of its yang contracting qualities, the gums as well as firming up the teeth, preserving the exterior and the interior of the teeth. There are also several 'health food' varieties of toothpaste based on bicarbonate of soda, being yang which are not as effective as sea salt, but far better than the regular shop varieties. Always choose a toothpaste with the minimum amount of chemicals having a yang type of base. Always brush the teeth in the direction of growth, preferably with a 'medium' quality toothbrush made out of a natural material like bristle. The longest time without food where the teeth and gums are at rest is at night, so always ensure the mouth is alkaline during this period. So, even if you do not use sea salt or a derivative to clean your teeth, at least, rinse your mouth with a solution of sea salt and water as suggested above. Particularly if you have any problems in this area.

Fluoride and Cancer

Fluoride, a compound of fluorine, was discovered to strengthen tooth enamel and prevent caries and is now a popular additive in many commercial toothpastes. This is a convenient method to counteract the effects of sugars and junk food, however one extreme cannot not be cancelled out by another without a price. There have been several studies, notably in New Zealand that there is an increased risk of cancer where there is the fluoridation of water supplies, possibly suggesting that fluoride is carcinogenic. This is probably due to the chemical cocktail overload as well.

If the teeth have to be filled, steer clear of or change amalgam fillings, because they contain mercury which is a very poisonous substance, known to disrupt the central nervous system, circulation, respiration and linked to memory loss. Even though more expensive, there are filling materials like composite resin and even gold which are non toxic and inert, allowing the chi to flow more readily into the teeth, whereas amalgam besides being toxic, negatively interferes with the energy polarity of mouth.

The use of natural chewing gum is very good for the gums and teeth, as well a method of cleaning teeth whilst on the move. However avoid commercial 'sugar free' gums as the artificial sweeteners are detrimental to the teeth, gums and the organism. When and if you can buy gum from a health store it will pay dividends in the long run.

Exercise

Surprisingly enough there are exercises to ensure that the gums and teeth stay strong and healthy, obviously accompanied by the afore mentioned guidelines. First thing in the morning brush the teeth with the relevant yang medium preferably a derivative of sea salt.

1) Then gently click the upper and lower teeth together, thirty two times. Like all things it will take a bit of practice to keep the jaws aligned. This has two main effects, firstly it encourages blood and chi to flow in these areas, strengthening the gums and the teeth. Secondly it also has a resonating, therapeutic effect to clear the brain, after its nightly yinnisation and rest.

2) Finally use the tongue to massage the gums by circling it around the outside of the teeth, with the tip of the tongue pressed firmly upwards, right up to where the top and bottom lip meet the upper and lower jaws, in as large a circle as possible. Then do the inside of the teeth pressing as much of the tongue, as is practicable against the inner parts of the upper and lower teeth, right up to and along the gums as well. Do in sets of thirty-two, sixteen times around the outer sides, followed by sixteen cycles for the inner areas. This has many benevolent side effects besides helping to keep the teeth clean. It massages the gums and teeth as well as exercising the whole of the tongue at the same time, which is related to the heart energy. This encourages a healthy flow of blood and chi to the area; also this method increases saliva which helps to maintain the desired alkaline presence in the mouth.

The teeth, as I wrote earlier, are dependent on the quality of the internal energy as well, therefore Tai Chi and the following Chi Kungs will be beneficial from Part 3 - 1), 2), 4), 5), 6), 7), 8) & 9) finished off by 1a) and 1b). These Chi Kungs tone and balance the chi, including the 'kidney essence' which is responsible for the bones as well as the structure of the teeth.

Always check with a medical practitioner if you are going to take herbal remedies whilst taking prescribed medicines.

PART THREE

The Science of The Inner Breath - Chi Kung

Yin and Yang and Chi

Here follows a practical guide to building and conserving the internal energy, the 'chi' of the body, in order to stimulate, circulate, balance, build and store this life force in a practical 'Western' manner; to promote, maintain and extend a healthy centred life. The world is made up of and ordered by opposite tendencies such as hot-cold, push-pull, young-old, tall-short, rich-poor, neutron-electron, inner-outer and so forth, which is evident but not usually recognised. These opposites happen at every level from the formation of a galaxy right down to the atom. The Taoist sages in ancient China adopted this law of opposites into their philosophy, science and medicine. They considered that their Universe was made of a life force which in its expanding phase was called 'yang' and when it reached its limit it changed into a contracting force, entitled 'yin'. The interacting combination of these two parts of the one force being responsible for all manifestation. This life force or chi has differing fractal levels, all obeying the law of yin and yang. Although from the same source, there was a Tao or great energy of the Universe responsible for all matter, including the planets, Earth energy and last but not least the yin yang components of the human, animal and plant kingdom. The superficial result of this unseen life force is the material world and all its variety. The Chinese character for yin indicates the dark side of a mountain with the yang being the sunny side.

The Taoists, to promote an understanding of creation, exploited this natural law, reasoning, like Descartes in the West, that the smaller cannot create the greater, therefore to understand the greater one should study the smaller.

Ursa Major

Two and a half thousand years before the birth of Christ, the Taoists observed that the North Star, was circumnavigated by the seasonal pointer of the seven stars of Ursa Major, apparently sitting statically in the opposite polar segment of the Heavens to the Earth. This gave rise to their reasoning, that by the law of opposites, the source of Universal energy came from that area. In 1993 this was confirmed by astronomers who discovered by way of the Hubble telescope, in its space orbit four hundred miles above the Earth, that the area behind Polaris was the birthplace of the Big Bang.

This principle of opposites evolved into discovering that if there is an outer breath, there must be an inner human microcosmic version. This internal life force was also called chi. The Chinese dictionary defines chi as breath, air or a gas deriving from the character signifying the dawn mist rising off a mountain, symbolising it as a manifestation of the eternal creative spirit. This science of inner breath was named Chi Kung, in Pinyin Chinese it is romanized as qigong, the word kung or gong signifying the working or practice of chi or qi. There are many types of Chi Kung which fall into two categories, the inner, 'nei', or outer 'wài' forms.

The most effective and superior are the internal Chi Kungs, collated and passed down by the Tai Chi masters of the Yang Family. These nei kung breathing exercises have been practised for three thousand years and were perfected by the Taoists of Wudang Mountain monastery in central China near Xían, an ancient capital of China famous for the tombs of the terracotta warriors. The Yang family hermetically improved the potential of these disciplines in both the martial and health spheres.

Obviously there are many stages of yin and yang just as night evolves into day and vice versa, represented by the Tai Chi Diagram, yin representing the black segment balanced by the white part of the yang half. If the chi goes out of kilter one of the segments would be larger than the other. The aim of Chi Kung is to harmonise the chi into homeostasis because if the chi is either too yin or yang it causes dis'ease'. All the organs, immune function, the senses, the central and sympathetic nervous systems, brain and body functions are supported by this internal energy. Therefore if this energy is disturbed it will cause disharmony. Even the English word heal is derived from 'whole' so when one is not 'whole' one is unwell.

Celestial Stems and Feng Shui

These concepts were born out of Taoist alchemy influencing many other philosophical systems such as Tai Chi Chuan and Feng Shui. The Taoist Masters developed a system of cyclical correspondences, the Wu Hsing, based on similar concepts to the Western Four Elements of the ancient Greeks. The Wu Hsing are the Five Stages of Changes of energy (fig.11) which tabulate the level of the chi in the seasons and the human body. Briefly the five stages of terrestrial chi are Fire, representing the restful heat of summer giving rise to the ripening bounty of the Earth stage of late summer. This transforms into the harvesting period of Autumn representing the closing or contracting level, symbolized by the cold compact structure of Metal. This announces the quiet, dark, fallow state of winter which in Chinese alchemy is epitomised by Water. In turn transmuting into the next stage of Wood being the new growth of spring with its inevitable return of rising energy when plants and trees begin their expansive plane fed by water and sun. Thus the cycle finishes its annual procession with Wood feeding the Fire of Summer.

Every element has a correspondence to an internal organ. Thus Fire represents the heart and mind, Earth is linked to the stomach, whereas Metal is the element associated with the lungs, Water is connected to the kidneys and Wood is allied to the Liver. These observations are still practised medically and have valid health ramifications. The Wu Hsing, referred to as the 'Five Elements' represent the energy potential not the literal meaning. For example summer is hot and linked to the heat of the sun in high summer, so when the body burns with a fever it is too yang therefore one has too much fire chi and so forth.

The Taoists incorporated these principles of the Wu Hsing into their Chi Kung linking Fire to consciousness, representing the active mind. So when the mind or mind's eye is focused at the level of the Chihoi (CV.6) (*fig.14*) which is the frontal aspect of the psychic center called the Tan Tien (dantián) it would generate 'heat'. This metaphorical concentration of the Fire of the mind when situated under the Water potential of the kidneys would transform its essence which was called jing. Jing is the instinctual yet unconscious generative potential of the body, called pre-birth chi. This form of meditative Chi Kung is the first stage of transmuting

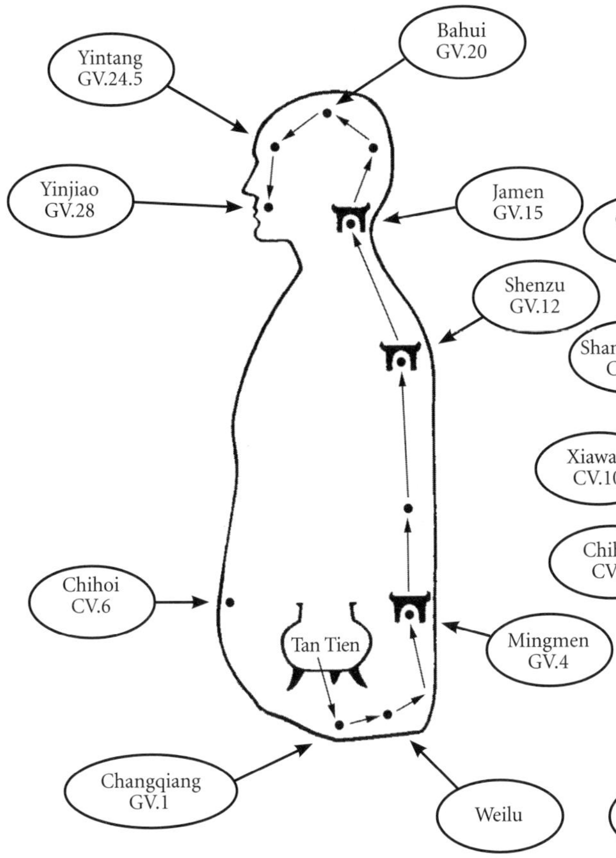

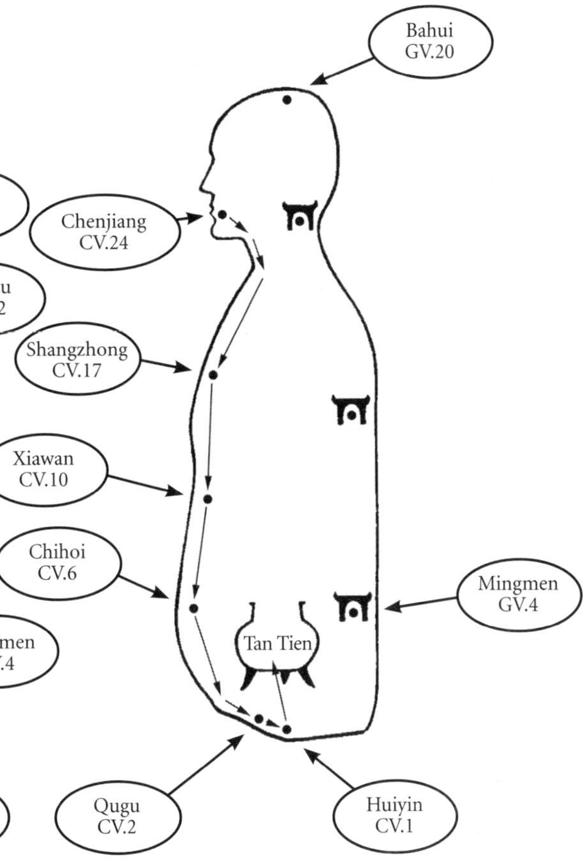

Figure 14a: The salient points of the Dumo Meridian and the direction of chi flow in the 'microcosmic' orbit.

Figure 14b: The salient points of the Renmo Meridian and the direction of chi flow in the 'microcosmic' orbit.

the inner life force into a tangible energy to enhance health, art, martial arts etc..

Red and Ancient China

This focusing of Fire under Water 'heats' the Water chi into an internal 'steam' or breath which is then conserved in the Tan Tien for later use. The Chinese characters for Tan Tien indicate a 'red or cinnabar field', hiding the deeper meaning of a cultivated place of heated yang energy. This red colour being an exoteric symbol of the esoteric life force, 'nei chi'. Derivatives of this spiritual symbolism crept into all walks of life consciously or not. Red cinnabar is the mineral ore of mercury and this red mercuric sulphide was used to paint artifacts including the renowned Chinese red lacquer called t'i hung. Also I suspect unknowingly, Chairman Mao adopted red, for his famous little book and the national flag.

Li Shao Chun, a Taoist alchemist of the second century B.C. advocated that the first step to achieving immortality was the metamorphosis of cinnabar by dedicating prayers to Tsao Chün, the Furnace Prince, who would help the adept to transmute mercury into gold. Here mercury carries the same meaning for both the Chinese and Western alchemists. In the West,

Mercury was not only a metal, the Roman messenger of the gods and a planet, but came to represent the arcane substance from the Holy Grail itself. In other words 'mercury' was a collective metaphor for the unconscious, lying in the manner of speech below matter or consciousness whilst gold was the result of the transmutation of this arcane element. The gold exemplifying the goal of the quest, being wholeness.

The Tan Tien, as well as acting as the cauldron of transformation, is also where the surplus chi can be stored. When the cauldron is heated, the chi, figuratively speaking, can spill out and down to the Huiyin (CV.1) (*fig.14*), the center of the perineum. Where it can be raised up into the Dumo channel which when correctly opened allows chi to ascend this meridian up the spine to the crown of the head, through the Baihui (GV.20). Ready for its descent through the Renmo for another firing at the Tan Tien. Every cycle making the unconscious chi more conscious. Jing being the alchemical spirit trapped in matter. The Baihui is linked to the 'Niewan' a Chinese term indicating a 'palace of enlightenment', known as Nirvana in Buddhism. The chi can then be tempered in a variety of ways to improve health, conduct martial skills and finally, for some, to achieve a spiritual oneness. (*See* Chi Kung exercises below).

The Source of Chi in the East and West

Jing is the pre birth or generative force, titled 'kidney (adrenal) essence' which for the Taoists was a life force emanating from the Nothing of Emptiness, Wu, before the Something of Manifestation, suggesting a pre-emptive energy from the time space void, responsible for all creation. It manifests itself through different mediums in different proportions of yin and yang to produce the plethora of Creation designated by Lao Tsu, as the 'ten thousand things'. This has a similar concept to the zero point energy of 'over unity' which is termed an 'esoteric force' by modern science. Over unity is the phrase for the phenomenon where one can extract more energy from matter i.e. anti-matter, than is put in. The Western Alchemists considered a substance known as phlogiston to be the hidden fire at the center of matter which was dismissed for centuries as hocus pocus until now, with the advent of the quantum theory and nuclear sciences.

The inner life force which the Chinese called jing can be compared in Western biology, despite the different perspective of Chinese medicine, to the variety of hormonal secretions, especially those deriving from the adrenal glands which are responsible for synthesising many of the body's hormones, including the androgens and the oestrogens. Jing naturally transmutes into chi which is responsible for and underlies the biological and chemical reactions that Western science and medicine has adopted in its understanding of the mind and body.

Neils Bohr - Quantum Yin Yang

Neils Bohr was a danish physicist who developed quantum mechanics in the 1920s, which is only now being studied and understood. He also launched the process of splitting the atom which lead to the atom bomb. He cited that, *"If you do not find the Quantum field surprising then you do not understand it"*. On his coat of arms, he placed the Yin Yang symbol and the latin phrase *"Contraria sunt Complimentia"* (opposites are complementary).

Chi, Hormones and DNA

The steroid hormones are essential for life, being the male and female hormones of reproduction. The adrenal medulla is composed of embryonic cells originating from the neural crest, pinched off during the formation of the neural tube of an embryo which is the fetal precursor of the spinal cord. The gonads (male testes and female ovaries) of both the men and women are embryonic cousins, having been attached to the adrenal glands of the fetus. They migrate downwards to differentiate into the appropriate sex of each individual at around six or seven months after conception. However bizarre a science, it is now possible for clinicians to extricate the ovarian follicles from a female fetus which can be fertilised in order to produce human beings.

The Chinese Masters regarded the mind and body as the result of the differing levels of chi with the physical attributes of the mind and the body being concrete manifestations of this life force. Western science discarded the concept of an inner soul in the eighteenth century at the advent of the so-called age of enlightenment, taking anatomy as its basis for understanding the mind and body. This became the new method of classifying the various physical phenomena, in a snap shot fashion ignoring the ebb and flow of a separate life force. The difference between the Eastern and Western science being purely conceptual. Western science could be described as observing the natural functions of the body as a compilation of millions of still photographs whereas the East saw the organism as a continuous film. To understand the plot one does not need to see each frame individually. Thus hormones would be the result of chi which in reality have the same function, although from a different perspective.

Centuries ago the Taoists proclaimed that the generative potential, 'jing' was passed on to offspring solely by way of the mother. This theory is similar to the present Western notion of the mitochondrial DNA which are the microscopic 'powerhouses' that provides a cell's energy. These cells have their own separate DNA strand, having been discovered by modern geneticists to be passed on only by the mother.

Stem Cells

These are the manifestation of the power of chi stored in a cell. Until stem cells are understood from the perspective of internal energy, the research will be of no long term value to humankind. However this layer of science is peeling away the purely mechanical and anatomical view of the human condition which has to end up with the energetic viewpoint of the organism.

One Ova, Billions of Spermatozoa and Chi

However, whichever perspective is taken, the potential of the gonads is enormous. A healthy male can produce 300,000,000 - 400,000,000 spermatozoa in one orgasm, and assuming a conservative estimate of a twenty year period of potency would allow a man to produce one, thousand, four hundred and fifty six billion sperm (1,456,000,000,000,) each capable of producing a female or a male with the same capability. Yet women produce both the male and the female out of one ova. Jing, being the generative essence, is passed on only by the female and is the mother of chi. This precious essence with its fantastic capability was the arcane elixir for the Taoist Alchemists. However incredulously, they came to this knowledge, confirmed by Western science, it is immaterial. Fact is fact, there is written proof that they conceived their process of harnessing and exploiting this extraordinary life producing substance in the second millennia B.C. before the tools of modern microbiology.

Comparable spiritual procedures are to be found elsewhere. It is not a coincidence that there are vows of celibacy and silence in many religious orders around the world, consciously or not acting as hermetic methods of containing this internal energy. The hermetic value of the inner strength being transformed by prayers and devotions. This being another way of confining this internal power within the body and by concentrated mental and physical strivings of one sort or another, the internal energy was transformed by the diverse devotions and vocal expressions, static or otherwise.

Transmutation of Chi in Mozart and Morris Dancers

These practices are to be found throughout the world including the sung mantras and sutras of the East, along with the celebrated 'A-u-m', where the 'Au' vibrates the lower psychic centers and the 'Um' the upper. Similarly the ancient Latin Mass included incantations like the Gregorian Chant which were based upon Judaic and Arabic sung prayers, intending to engender this uplifting effect.

The Native Americans and Aboriginal rituals have dances and songs for certain seasons and rites with like intentions of transmuting the basic human instincts in order to raise awareness of the spiritual destiny of man. This process, with a little discernment, can be seen in folk dancing from all countries, like the English Morris dancers and their maypole rituals. The tapping of clogs represent the beat of the Earth's horizontal force being formalized by dancing gestures creating a set of spiralling interwoven patterns formed around the maypole, being the upright symbol of masculine heavenly power. The performers acting out a cosmic dance with the intention of marrying these opposites for the benefits of the people and their land, an English version of Feng Shui.

All of these methods stimulate, circulate and raise the energy around the mind and body. Research carried out in the UK discovered that certain 'classical' music like Mozart, can improve mental concentration and learning. Children became more responsive and receptive when Mozart's music was played in the background during lessons. Some surgeons have classical music piped into the operating theatres as they find this music relaxing, but sharpening the necessary senses of the whole team during surgery. Mozart was introduced to Freemasonry by his Masonic father and it is considered by some scholars that all his music is based on numerical themes from the Kabalah. This Jewish book of mysticism is a corner stone of many Western clandestine orders. Newton spent more time studying it than studying orthodox science. The Magic Flute, his last major work is such an example, being based on a beat of seven.

Each of these, although from distinct cultures, employed the penetrating ability of the musical resonance allied with disciplines to achieve the same goal, consciously or not, of causing the lower pre-birth energy of pro-creation to metamorphosise into spirit.

Prana and Chi

In Kundalini (serpent power) Yoga, the prana or chi is raised up in a vertical plane and transmuted through the seven chakras by certain yogic disciplines. Initiated at the lowest chakra of mulhadara (earth chakra - Huiyin - CV.1) in the genital area up to the sahasrara (thousand lotus petals/nirvana - Bahui - GV.22) at the top of the head.

Jung and Chi

Professor Carl Jung developed a process of individuation, independently discovering an eclectic procedure of finding wholeness or the center of one's being, which he called the Self. He outlined this process to involve archetypes being common to all cultures and religions basically identifiable as a Good God, The Devil, Female or Male Deities and a human hero on a quest. The method he developed elucidates all the various systems observing that the symbols from each culture meant in essence the same thing, simply a person striving for self knowledge by making conscious, the mysterious archetypes of the unconscious.

His version of individuation is fulfilled by becoming truly aware and absorbing the instinctual energy of the archetypes which are the unconscious parts of the psyche, projected out onto matter. In this way we meet our unconscious as fate, because the unconscious, yin elements of our psyche naturally seek out their yang counterparts in the outer world of events and experiences.

Unfortunately when we meet such outer events as the result of unconscious projections, it is usually unpleasant. But if one can reflect on the seemingly dank, damp inner world of the unconscious, it can prevent unnecessary hardships, thus turning fate into destiny. Reflection being the way to seal in the energy of the projections, creating an inner heat of anguish, being transformed by the honest fire of conscious thought into an inner strength of clarity. This metamorphosis of our own unconscious, enriching and enlarging our consciousness.

Thoughts, written and spoken words have hidden power distinctly confirmed by their ability to teach, control or influence. (*See also* Stress Section or *Refer to* ***Time for a Change***). Individuation is a process that draws out the unconscious elements of the psyche making them allies, as opposed to fatalistic tools of learning and destiny. Below the ego consciousness lies the shadow being the same gender as the person.

The next level is the contra-sexual soul which Professor Jung called the animus in women being masculine and the feminine anima in men. This inner soul when accepted not only allows an individual to have a positive relationship with a partner, but opens the door to the center of the psyche which Jung called the Self, representing wholeness of the human, being the same gender as the person, thus when the positive yang and negative yin energies are in harmony.

Jung noticed that the process of individuation is usually kick started by an outer traumatic event, often accompanied by a flood of dreams from the unconscious which if accepted as autonomous aspects of the psyche will commence the inner dialogue and 'alchemical' journey towards wholeness.

Whatever process is adopted the archetypes will always manifest themselves, as Jung discovered, appertaining to the culture and origin of the psyche concerned. Whichever scheme, is used it must never be forced or induced chemically by drugs and so forth, but must be a natural process.

Taoist Fire and Chi

The Taoist Fire of the mind in Chi Kung is associated to the hypothalamus with its brother of the pituitary gland. Even in modern Chinese medicine, which is a blend of Traditional Chinese Medicine and Western medicine, it is accepted that the Baihui (GV.20) *(fig.14)* stimulates this area of the mid-brain, the Baihui means the place of a 'Hundred Convergences'. The inner eye of the pineal, is also stimulated by way of the Yintang (GV.24.5)*(fig.14)*, which is the site of the outer aspect of the 'Third Eye' of Eastern culture, the Yintang is an acupoint situated on the forehead at the glabella, just above and between the eyebrows.

This 'third eye' spot on the forehead is a locus stimulated in many creeds, where this region is activated in the Jewish religion by attaching a prayer apparatus and wailing. In Islam this area is tapped on the ground whilst praying towards Mecca. The Lamist Buddhists used to trepan this sector, in young religious acolytes, by taking a slither of bamboo and gently piercing through the skull at the Yintang. Then inserting the bamboo tool to the required depth to arouse this segment of the brain, in order to encourage second sight for spiritual purposes.

Hormones and The Third Eye

In Western medicine this median area of the brain, the Eastern third eye, controls the hormonal glands. Also overseeing directly some hormonal secretions such as adrenaline, noradrenaline, and the growth hormones of the androgens and oestrogens; as well as regulating body heat, wakefulness and sleep, organising metabolism, sexual differentiation, desires and drives of life, monitoring appetites for food, drink and sex, as well as controlling blood pressure and the autonomic nervous system including neurotransmitters, neuromodulators and neurohormones. This central area also inter-reacts with many other parts of the brain. It appears that both the East and West, although using different terminology, acknowledge this part of the anatomy as an exceedingly important structure of the organism.

Sex and Chi

Chi Kung has some interesting offshoots, one of which entered the realm of increasing sexual potential. Here I shall only cover the salient aspects relating to this subject. A man can drastically drain his life force by excessive release of sperm which is a physical manifestation of chi, being the male evolutionary mechanism of ensuring future offspring. It is chi that creates the sperm, the firmness of an erection and the mechanics of ejaculation. Healthy chi ensures potency and fertility, the reverse is obviously true, but can be enhanced by reducing stress, practicing Chi Kung and eating a balanced diet as laid out in this book.

A balanced sex life will not do any harm to a man's internal energy. The body will give out plenty of warning signals such as tiredness, unusual or continual bouts of illness, pulled muscles, strained tendons, bad backs, pains in joints and so forth. If the chi supply is exhausted it will effect the energy fed into the meridians which sustains the homeostasis of the body including the immune function. Jing chi is naturally converted into chi on a daily basis, therefore if one burns up more energy than is readily available, the body draws chi from other areas, hence illness or injury is more likely to occur.

Sexuality is certainly not simply about sensual gratification, as caring for a partner with feeling is more appreciated and important than sexual athletics. A caring sharing attitude will help engender a stable relationship, adding to the well being of any couple. There are now plenty of books on mutually enhancing sexual pleasure. Both men and women can deplete their jing chi, by general stress, prolonged illness, pathogens, pollution, poor diet, excessive exercise and especially strenuous mental exertion; as most of these are almost inevitable, engaging in regular Chi Kung and or Tai Chi will build a reserve for that inevitable rainy day, thus storing, preserving and building on original jing chi.

Childbirth and Chi

Women need healthy amounts of jing for childbirth which depletes this female pre-birth chi, but an average woman has more than enough for these miracles of nature. The female does not lose any chi during a normal sex life, which can actually stimulate the conversion of jing into chi. If a woman does not have children, the excess chi, if not addressed, can lead to physical and psychological problems, as the chi has an inherent intent of unconscious self manifestation albeit disturbing or aesthetic. Childbirth is often replaced by alternative offspring such as a career, creative endeavors, business ventures and so forth, this being more common today in this overcrowded world, as long as it is in control and conscious. Chi Kung and Tai Chi, besides improving health generally, are an excellent natural way of ameliorating, mutually, sexual gratification and potency for both men and women, as well as ensuring healthy offspring.

Chi as an Investment

Chi Kung is an effective tried and tested way of adding to the original finite amount of jing that is passed on to each child by the mother. One can imagine chi to be like an investment of money deposited in a bank with each person being born with a certain inherited sum passed on by the parents. Therefore if one inherits the usual healthy amount and leads a normal lifestyle, it will be used up accordingly giving rise to an average constitution and life span. However if a person leads a life of extremes, unfortunately his or her chi will be squandered leading to illness and possibly a premature end. Please bear in mind the Chinese saying that one still has a chance if one has one breath left in the body.

On the other hand one can supplement the pre-birth chi, by the Chi Kungs laid out below or other disciplines which can increase the capital sum allowing one to live a full life off the interest and less of the capital, until destiny calls. This methodology is the secret of the celebrated, wholesome longevity of the Taoists and others.

There are a plethora of Chi Kungs, of which I shall explain ten distinct methods which improve mind and body. One must not do any circulating or advanced Chi Kungs when one is ill or recovering from an illness. This applies especially to women who should abstain from Chi Kung during menstruation. Menstruation is a natural way of discharging toxins from the body. Also Chi Kung can drain the chi away from the natural healing process of an organ or an area or the body which may be in a state of self-cleansing. So if one circulates chi during these unbalanced periods, one could re-absorb the toxins which should be discharged. One has to wait until well before doing or resuming the more involved Chi Kungs.

Inner and Outer Breath

The backbone of Taoist Chi Kung incorporates reverse or pre-birth breathing, so named because it simulates the abdominal 'breathing' during the ingestion of nutrients that the fetus receives from the mother in the womb. This is where the belly is drawn in and up in the same fashion as in the womb state, reproduced in the reverse breathing techniques of Chi Kung, clinically referred to as antidromic breathing.

All Taoist breathing techniques use reverse breathing at their core. Research in Japan and France showed that this system of respiration is ten times more effective at absorbing O_2 and displacing CO_2 than regular breathing. It also acts as an abdomino-thoraic pump, that is, it assists the dark venal blood filled with CO_2 and toxins up to the heart and lungs for displacement more effectively. Reverse breathing massages the viscera and above all animates the pre-birth chi of the adrenals and the gonads of both women and men. During reverse breathing, the naturally raised testicles and the female ovaries are activated, as well as supporting the rotation of chi in the Dumo and Renmo channels, (*fig.14*) referred to as the micro cosmic orbit.

Chi Kung is a specific procedure of energy conversion, at the beginning one might not notice any specific sensations, which can be felt in a variety of ways such as tingling, itching, heat, static, magnetic fields and so forth. Primarily the sensations can be negligible and awareness of them is unnecessary because it is enough just to visualise that the chi is circuiting in a certain way, which will have the desired effect. Chi will naturally follow the intent of the mind however slight, the amount, flow and sensations will increase with practice. Every person will feel their chi in different ways which is unwittingly experienced during illness when the chi is out of harmony, expressing its discord, as flushes, chills, fevers, hot and cold sensations, aches and pains, general itching and so forth. For example an everyday occurrence is to scratch one's head over a problem, which is in fact stimulating the flow of chi to the brain just as rubbing an area of the body after a knock is soothing.

Only perform these breathing exercises when feeling well, in clean, pollution free environments, away from drafts and the wind, ensuring not to loose body heat. Do not carry out when the mind is an altered state due to extreme moods, drugs or alcohol. It is advisable to leave a space of at least thirty minutes or so either side of carrying out Chi Kung, therefore do not eat or drink excessive amounts of liquid or cold drinks. Steer clear of physical exertion, avoid bathing, showers and going to the toilet during this period. Chi can be disturbed when the internal organs are active in digestion or when the heart and lungs are agitated.

Right Time for Chi Kung

Chi Kung is more beneficial when carried out early mornings, in a natural familiar and harmonious situation. It is acceptable to perform in the early evening, but not too late because the body's chi becomes steadily more yin after midday. This is a natural mechanism which permits the system to rest and refresh itself during its nightly yin phase. Yin rests and dilates whereas yang contracts and excites, this the reason for the general custom for people to sleep at night and work during the day. If Chi Kung is carried out sensibly for twenty minutes or so, between the hours of 3.00 p.m. and 7.00 p.m. (UK/GMT or local solar time) when cyclical chi is charging the bladder and kidney meridians, it will also nourish the habitual and pre-birth chi of these organs.

An everyday, visual effect of chi is the humble yawn illustrated by the opening of the mouth caused as the yang chi descends from the head into the body, countered by the ascent of the yin chi at night and vice versa in the morning. This is a natural yet involuntary opening of the mouth expressing this interchange of energy. A simple aid to nocturnal restlessness is to concentrate on the feet which will aid any errant yang chi that may be trapped in the head, in order to calm and allow it to descend to its nightly home. This calming exercise can be assisted by deep breathing with the joined hands held over the Chihoi (CV.6), as in 1) below, allowing the chi to harmonise. Obviously this will not rid one of the cause of the unrest, but can give a welcome respite to the psyche, opening a timely window for reflection and a solution. The only way to truly deal with a problem is to face it openly and honestly because the cure always lies at the root, just as yang lies at the heart of yin and vice versa.

Chi Kungs are more potent at vitalising pre-birth chi, when 'post-birth' chi of nature is harmonious in the form of fresh healthy air, clean and moderate fluid intake, a balanced diet of 70% yang to 30% yin of natural foods (*See* Part 1 and the Yin Yang Diet).

One can directly absorb the 'post-birth chi' or energy of the sun which could be considered as residual ionic effects of the solar winds. When doing any 'in' yin breath imagine the energy of the sun being inspired into the lungs, then taken down into the Tan Tien along the Conception Vessel (*fig.14*). This is more efficacious when practised outside, early morning in a natural environment. This can accompany any Chi Kung done outside, even whilst lying or sitting in the sun.

Central Equilibrium

Standing or seated Chi Kungs must adopt the appropriate aspects of a Tai Chi term known as Central Equilibrium, which ensures the correct posture alignment of the necessary energy gates and channels. The principles of Central Equilibrium encourage chi to flow unimpeded through the various aspects of the meridians and organs.

Central Equilibrium is a term coined by the Tai Chi Masters, specifically attributed to Yang Cheng Fu, at the turn of the nineteenth century, who laid out the following principles to aid the transformation of jing into chi:-

Double Weighting

a) One should never 'double weight' when practicing Chi Kung, implying that 70% of the weight should always be on one foot or the other. Double weighting causes the chi to stagnate in the lower limbs effecting the distribution of chi throughout the whole body, in the same way a building is as secure as its foundations.

Also 70% of the weight of each foot must be positioned over the 'Bubbling Well Point', Yongquan, the spot on the pad of the foot (K.1) (*fig.15*) with the other 30% on the heel acting as a stabilizer. This 70-30 ratio applies to both the 'weighted' yang foot and the accompanying yin foot.

It also applies to the yang foot of both a front and a back stance (*fig.15*). This distribution of weight uses natural law being the root of the entire Chi Kung and Tai Chi stances. If this part securely adheres to the Earth and intermixes with the chi of the Earth, it helps safeguard

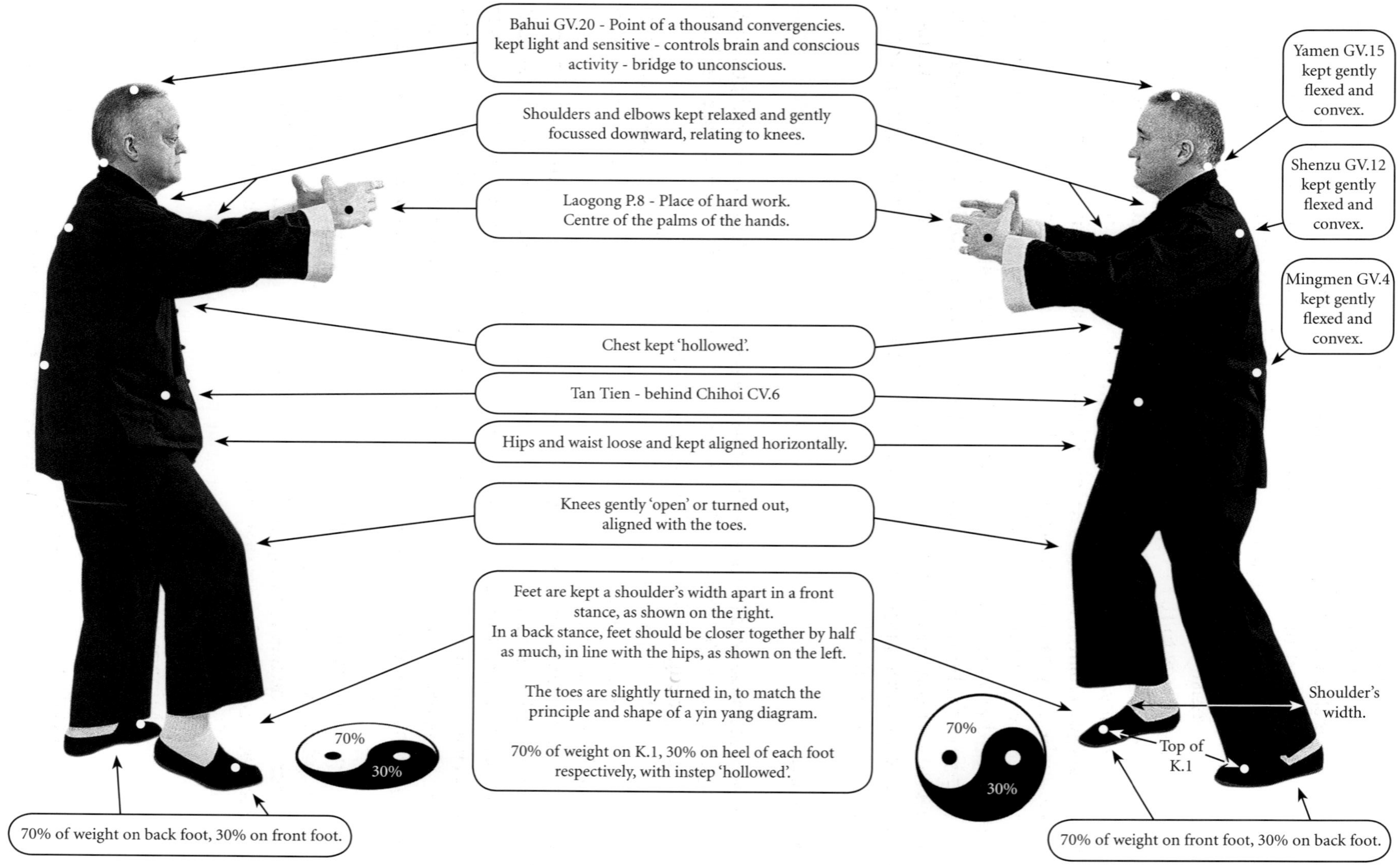

Figure 15: **Central Equilibrium** - The Essentials of the Tai Chi Chuan and Chi Kung posture.

Central Equilibrium. The Tai Chi classics refer to this loss of adhesion as floating. It is not by coincidence that this point is the start of the Kidney channel which is the home of pre-birth chi and when K1.is stimulated, it will engender more chi, therefore increasing stability.

The outer, convex part of a circle is yang and the inner concave aspect, yin. This law is evident in the humble, but essential inflated tyre of a vehicle. The outer yang side supported by the inner yin arc which holds the air. The same law of dynamics applies to chi, therefore a convex aspect will assist yang chi to flow in yang channels and the concave or hollow shape will encourage yin energy to run in yin channels. Therefore the feet should arc and cup the ground with the outer top sides of the foot making a convex yang curve, with the soles making a yin concave, always ensuring that K.1. is rooted. The toes must be kept relaxed and as straight as possible as many meridians terminate and begin at the ends of the feet.

Chi rises up the body naturally as we age, the higher the centre of gravity the nearer death. Therefore if chi rises prematurely it indicates an unhealthy condition, this why the Tai Chi classics prescribe that one breaths with one's feet. Meaning one must keep the center of gravity in the middle of the body at the Tan Tien, with the feet yang and the head yin. Figuratively keeping the human centered between the forces of heaven and earth. In Complementary Medicine, there are observational techniques of where and how chi relates to a person, acting as an accurate visual method of instant diagnosis.

Correct Stance

b) Front stances are measured by the width of one's own shoulders. A back stance aligns both feet within a parallel corridor structured on the inside by the heel of the weighted, yang, back foot and by the outer edge of the hip of the yin leg (*fig.15*).

The feet of a front stance should trace the edge of an imagined Tai Chi Tu , that encloses every stance. The diameter should be equal to the width of one's own shoulders. (*fig.15*) with the toes of each foot being slightly turned in.

The knee of the yang, weighted, leg must be over the toes of the yang foot and the knee of the yin leg must be aligned with the toes of the yin foot. The knees of the legs should be subtly turned out with the toes gently pointing in, creating an inner concave and outer convex to the shape of the legs. An exaggerated version of this can be seen in the bowed legs of a cowboy. These parameters will encourage chi to flow in the yang outer sides of each leg and foot, returning up the inner, yin aspect of the leg. Diseases of the lower limbs, where chi flow has been inhibited by accident or illness brings about a yinnising of the legs, causing the knees to buckle in towards each other. This can be seen in so called motor nerve diseases like Multiple Sclerosis etc.. If a person naturally has feet that turn in, it indicates a yang constitution whereas if the feet turn out, it shows the person to be more yin. This is noticeable in very young children even before they walk, determining the type of constitution inherited from the parents.

Sacrum Plumb - Mingmen - Shenzou - Jamen

c) The hips and the pelvis must be kept in an horizontal plane which will prevent any scoliosis which is a lateral curvature of the spine. This is usually caused by a yin diet, bad comportment or one leg being longer than the other. This complaint can be helped in time with

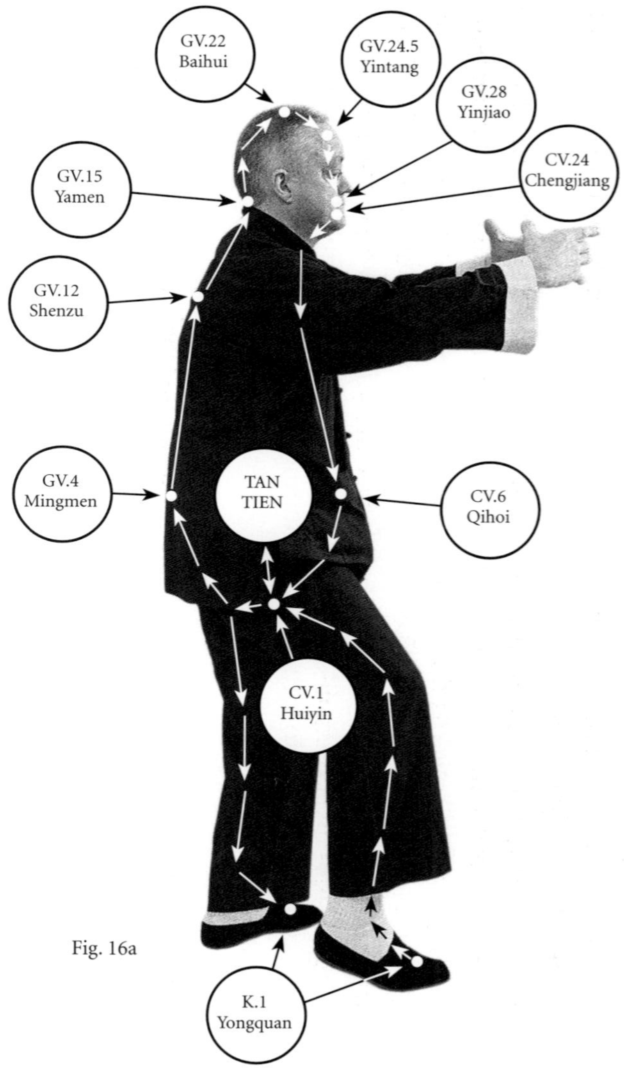

Fig. 16a

The flow of chi energy is designated by the white arrows in the figures.

The micro-cosmic orbit (left) is visualised with chi flowing from the Tan Tien, then down to the CV.1 (huiyin), up the spine through GV.4 (mingmen), GV.12 (shenzu), GV.15 (yamen), GV.22 (baihui), ending the yin in breath cycle at GV.28 (yinjiao) at the top lip. The out breath and yang cycle starts at CV.24 on the bottom lip, then descends the Conception Vessel terminating in the Tan Tien.

The macro-cosmic cycle (right) is a continuation of the above, where the yang out breath continues down from the CV.1 along the inside of both legs to K.1 on the pads of the feet. The yin in breath cycle starts at K.1 and the chi is drawn up and visualised up the outer median aspects of both legs to CV.1 (huiyin), then continues up the spine, over the head, ending at the top lip, GV.28. One full cycle being an out breath from CV.24 to K.1 and the in cycle from K.1 to GV.28.

Carry out either orbit in blocks of four. Please refer to Part 3 for full details.

Fig. 16a (left) is back stance where 70% of the weight is on the K.1 of the left and back leg.

Fig. 16b (right) is a forward stance where 70% of the weight is on the K.1 of the forward right leg.

One can carry out Chi Kung in either a back or a forward stance for ten minutes on each leg, starting with the weight on the left leg and the arms held high as in Fig. 16a, then changing the weight to the right leg and lowering the arms as in Fig.16b. Always stay relaxed and upright and use reverse breathing.

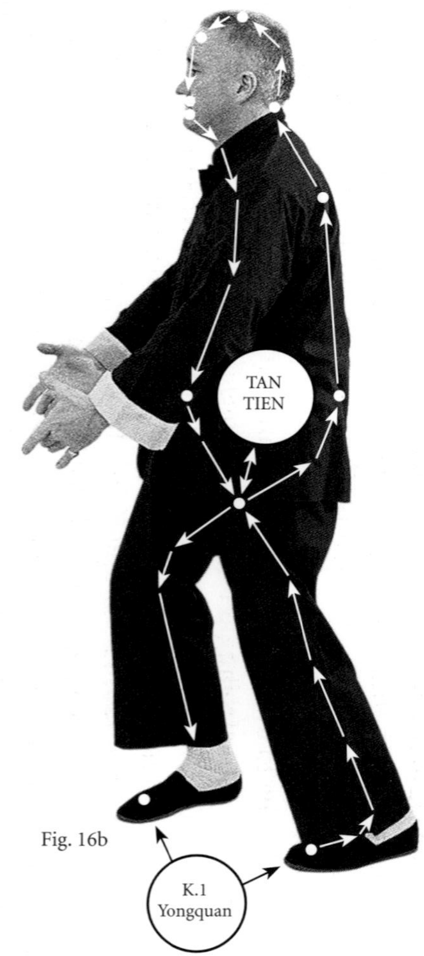

Fig. 16b

Figure 16a and 16b: **Micro/Macro Cosmic Breathing** - A schematic layout of the Micro and Macro cosmic orbits of chi circulation in Tai Chi Chuan and Chi Kung.

perseverance by Chi Kung and a balanced yin yang diet.

The Tai Chi classics state that 'Chi is stored in the spine' which means that the spine although kept vertical should have a gentle convex bow shape, accentuating the three main gates of chi amplification on the Dumo. The first is the Mingmen which stimulates kidney chi (GV.4) (*fig.15*), the next is the Shenzu (GV.12) located between the shoulder blades where the chi is fed to the arms and lastly the Jamen (GV.15) at the base of the hairline at the middle of the neck controlling the medulla oblongata and all its nerve and brain functions. The human Medulla Oblongata is the only example of any species on Earth to be directly over the spine and under the brain. The Tai Chi dictum 'the head must be kept light and sensitive' refers to the cranium summit point, the Baihui (GV.20), acting as though it was being pulled up vertically. This ethereal point is the bridge between the upward flow and descending arc of chi in the microcosmic orbit, invigorating the brain including the hypothalamus, the pituitary and the pineal glands. The Baihui is considered a point equated with Niewan or Nirvana, enlightenment. If the Yongquan (K.1) of the foot is well rooted and the Baihui is light and sensitive the body will be in harmony with the chi of Heaven and Earth.

Renmo and Dumo

d) The tongue is curled up to lightly touch the roof of the mouth, linking the Dumo and Renmo channels. The chin is kept in and the chest concave, at point Shanzong (CV.17) (2) on the sternum. This will balance the Fire and Water chi of the mind and body which is essential for health. The spine must be kept in a vertical line, with the sacrum vertically aligned with the spine. This helps connect the lower orbit of body chi at the gate of the Huiyin (CV.1).

Elbow and Shoulders

e) The arms must be relaxed and circular at all times. The elbows and shoulders must be kept low and loose, which helps to keep the chi centered at the Tan Tien, the frontal aspect being, the Chihoi (CV.6). If the shoulders are raised, the chi will float out of the body by way of the lung. This 'negative chi' raising of the shoulders can be seen in the disturbed chi of asthmatics or when people are frightened.

One should point the elbows downwards, in a rounded fashion, slightly away from the body to prevent any restriction of chi flow, ensuring the arms are not too close to the body. If the elbows are directed towards the knees in this way, it protects the floating ribs as well as helping to prevent the chi rising. When the shoulders and elbows are loose, relaxed and gently held in their sockets, the chi is more readily held at the Tan Tien preventing the energy from 'floating' besides preventing damage to the joints of the shoulders and the arms.

The Six Thieves

f) The wrists, ankles, knees, elbows, hips and shoulders must be kept relaxed and rounded, never held at acute, chi blocking angles. If these joints are tense or have sharp angles the chi is wasted or blocked.

Intention

g) Chi follows the mind and as the mind intent becomes stronger, the chi will become more powerful. The mind's eye is always focused at the Tan Tien. Every exercise being governed by the maxim, the mind moves the chi that moves the body. This seemingly impossible task is started by imagining or visualising that the chi is streaming in the desired manner through the body in specific ways. With practice, this inner ideation process of chi projection will pave the way to more involved patterns of chi circulation. After a while depending on the relative effort, as the thought chi becomes clearer, it will follow intent of the mind more easily. One must remain 'Sung' which loosely translated means to keep relaxed while maintaining all of the controlling parameters of Tai Chi's Central Equilibrium.

Supple Waist, Supple Chi

h) The Grand Master Yang Cheng Fu, declared '*Relax the waist. The waist rules the body*'. Here he means if the waist is rigidly held and not supple there will be no connection between upper and lower and the front and back. If the feet are not well rooted, the posture is insecure, preventing the waist from acting like the center of a wheel, being the central pivot which controls the chi between the upper and lower areas. This is accomplished firstly in a physical manner by ensuring that the Chi Kung adopts 'Chan Shu Jian from Tai Chi, the silk cocoon reeling' technique. This is where the body and the weighted leg turns inward, in a screw like fashion, down the relevant weighted leg driving the K.1 point of the foot into a sure footed stance. For example if the weight is forward in a front right stance, the waist should turn slightly towards the right foot without angling the hip out of its horizontal plane.

This process is then internalised by ideation where the chi does the 'turning' instead of the body which makes the outer twist almost imperceptible. The chi is directed outwards to the upper limbs and simultaneously down to K1. in two complimentary, spiralling actions, with the waist being the center of each twist of chi.

The relative success of developing chi will depend on the amount and quality of pre-birth chi available. The initial training of 'thought chi' is the inception of the legendary ability of the Yang Clan to levitate as well as being responsible for the unusual feats that these determined specialists were able to accomplish, perhaps exaggerated over time, but who knows. The Yang Family had a very private joke of duping the despotic Ching Rulers for two centuries. This was only made possible by these hidden secrets of mind intent which is how they retained their prowess and their necks intact for so long.

Movement Within Stillness and Stillness Within Movement

The ideal of Chi Kung is to achieve movement in stillness where the body is kept still permitting one to activate the jing into chi, fuse it with the mind then circulate it around the body, helped by adopting Central Equilibrium in a total intrinsic blend. The principles becoming second nature without having to focus on them at all, arriving at the point of an innate movement within stillness.

It is advisable to commence by doing Chi Kung rooted on the left leg first, and balance the exercise by doing the same amount on each leg, for example, start with ten minutes on the left leg then finish with ten minutes on the right leg, building up to one hour on each leg. The eyes should never be closed and should be kept slightly open without any particular focus, with the gaze lightly looking down the angle of the nose with the tongue resting gently on the soft palette, thus joining the Water and Fire channels of the back and front.

Pregnancy

N.B. When a woman becomes pregnant only do Chi Kung 1) below, because the baby is nurtured by the mother's chi. Chi Kungs 2) to 10) would adversely redirect the natural course of the mother's chi. It is very beneficial for mother and baby during pregnancy to practice relaxed deep breathing as in 1), sitting or lying down. It is also rewarding to perform gentle sets of Tai Chi without any mind focusing for the same reasons. The reverse breathing being changed to normal contractions of the abdomen.

Ten Basic Chi Kungs

Reverse Breathing

1). 'Reverse breathing' employs the abdominal muscles, whilst inhaling and exhaling. Reverse breathing is alluded to in the Tai Chi classic as 'fanning the fire', with the bellows of the abdomen because it excites the pre birth chi into conscious activity. The anal sphincter and the Huiyin (CV.1) the centre of the perineum, is held gently taut, pulled in and up as if preventing bowel and bladder motions. This anal tuck is retained in a relaxed manner for as long as possible during reverse breathing. This holding procedure will help prevent prostrate and testicular cancer in men, as well as being beneficial for any person with complaints in the area of the Huiyin, (CV.1, gathering place of yin). This process will strengthen and animate and exercise the pelvic floor muscle with chi. This complaint effects some women after childbirth or in later life when chi and muscle activity have waned.

On the 'in breath', being yin, the abdomen and diaphragm are drawn in and up, followed by the yang 'out breath' where the abdomen and diaphragm are extended out and down, without raising the ribcage. Always staying relaxed and calm, with the mind's eye held at the Tan Tien. This should be carried out in blocks of four. It can be done seated or standing and even lying on one's back with hands resting on the Chihoi (CV.6). When sitting, one can be in a crossed legged position, lotus, half lotus or sitting on one's calves, but preferably with the soles of the feet turned upwards. If one is unable to sit like this, it is fine to carry out this procedure on a chair with the soles of the feet placed flat down, the thighs parallel to the ground. The hands cupped together over the Tan Tien, the centre of each hand, the Laogong (P.8) over each other. The right hand covering the left at the Chihoi (CV.6) for women and the left over right for men. The hands may also be rested on the lap in the same order, with the thumbs facing forward and the little finger edge of the hands resting at the level of the Chihoi. Seated Chi Kung can be done discretely in public places or on journeys if the air and atmosphere are reasonable.

When standing (*fig.15*), it is more productive to keep the weight on one leg, a back stance being more potent than a front weighted posture. Nevertheless, a front weighted posture still has the edge over any 'double weighted' stances being the least effective as the chi of the lower

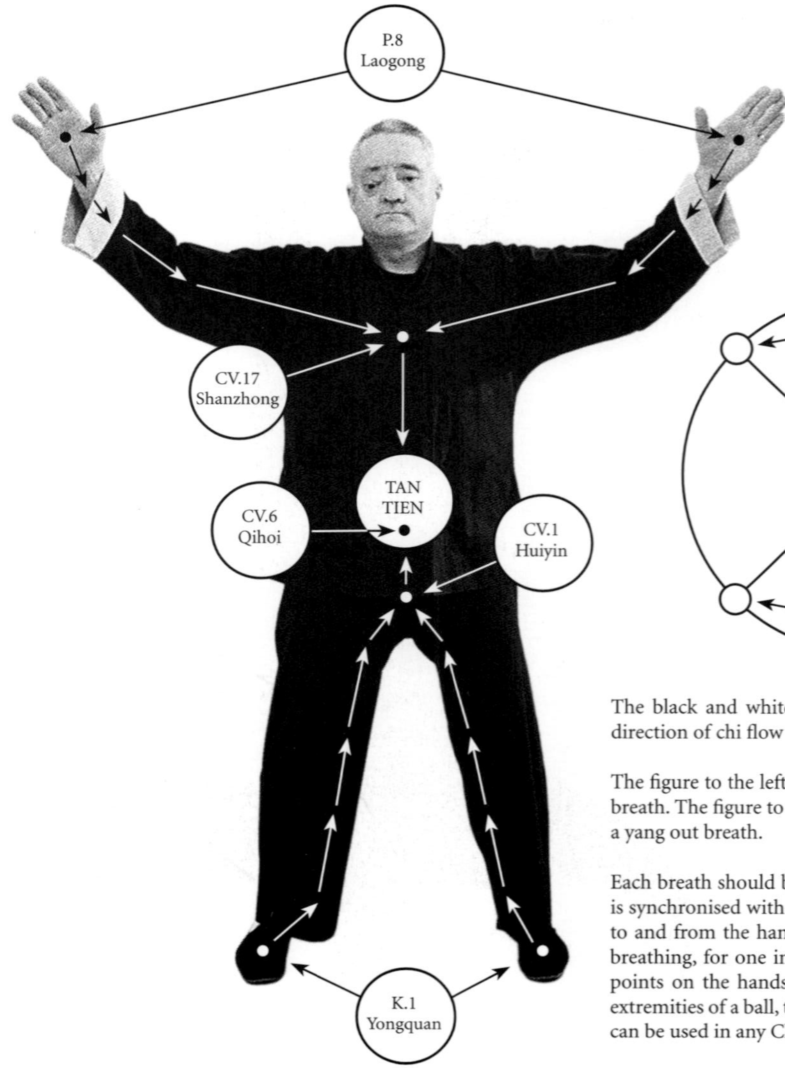

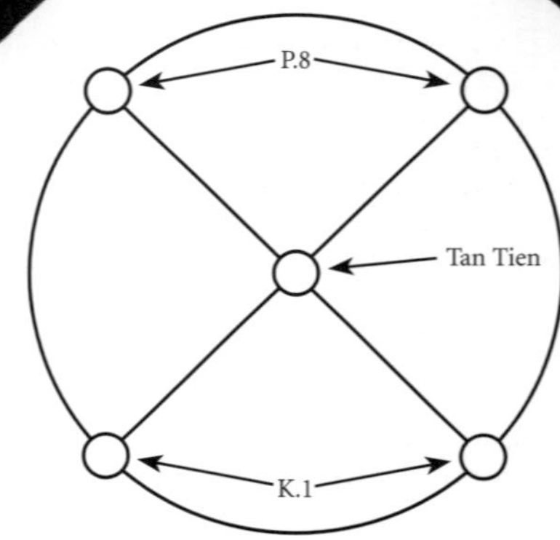

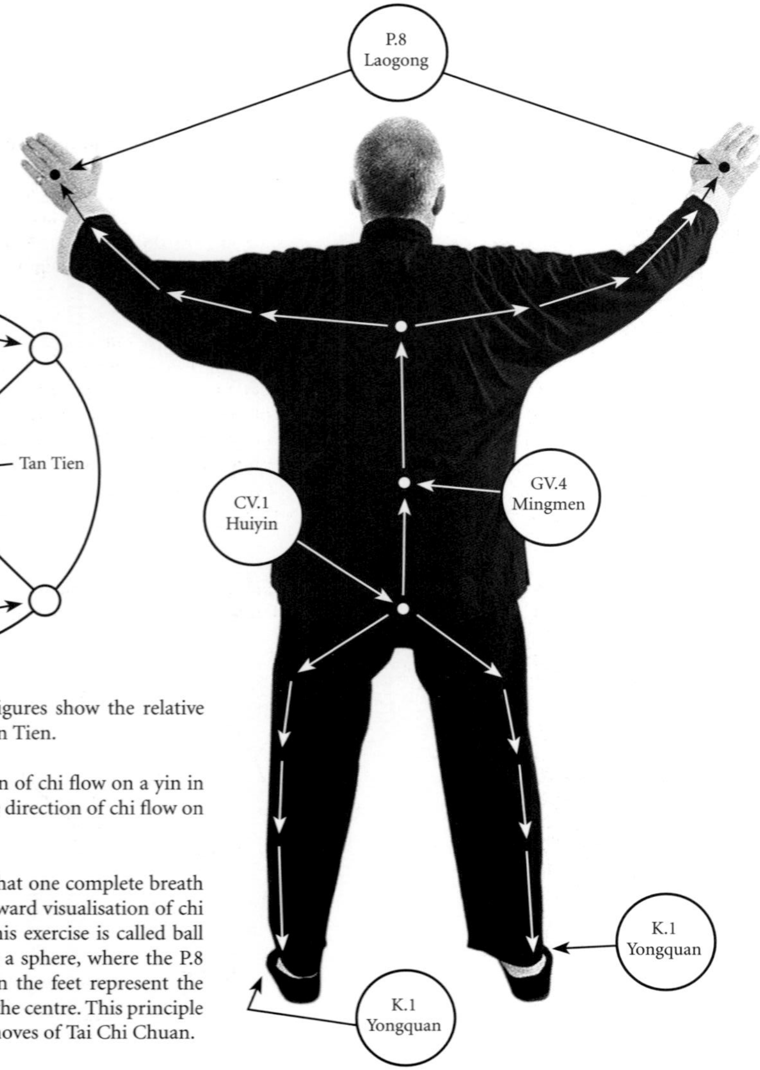

The black and white arrows in both figures show the relative direction of chi flow to and from the Tan Tien.

The figure to the left shows the direction of chi flow on a yin in breath. The figure to the right shows the direction of chi flow on a yang out breath.

Each breath should be coordinated so that one complete breath is synchronised with one outward or inward visualisation of chi to and from the hands and the feet. This exercise is called ball breathing, for one imagines that one is a sphere, where the P.8 points on the hands and K.1 points on the feet represent the extremities of a ball, the Tan Tien being the centre. This principle can be used in any Chi Kung or in the moves of Tai Chi Chuan.

Figure 17: **Ball Breathing** - A schematic picture of ball breathing and the flow of chi energy for Tai Chi Chuan and Chi Kung.

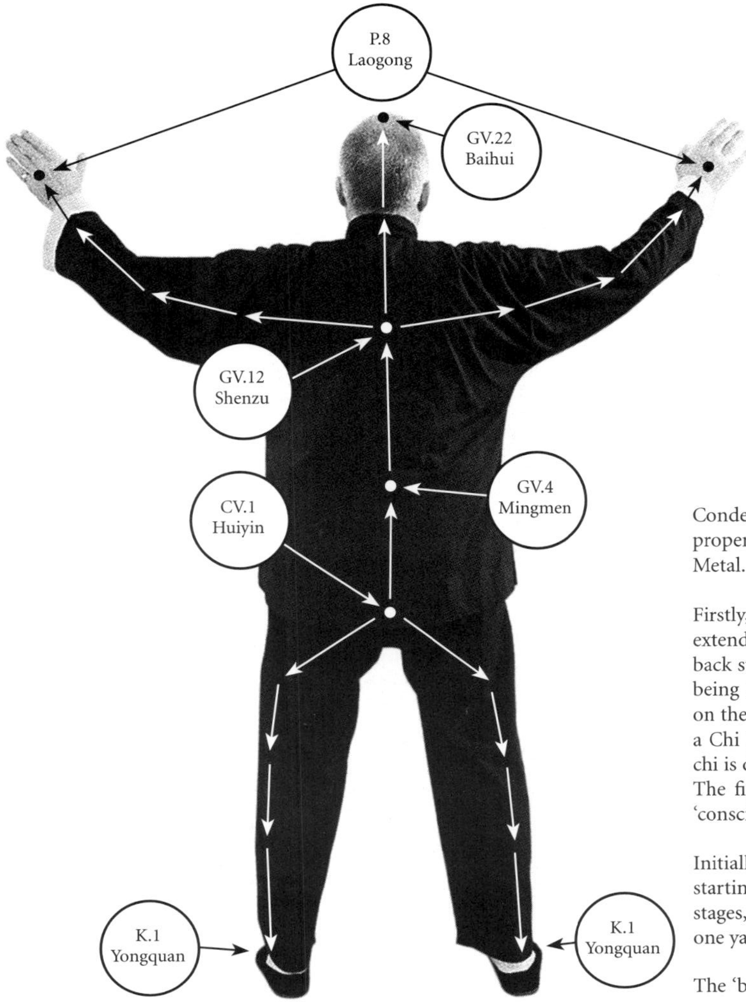

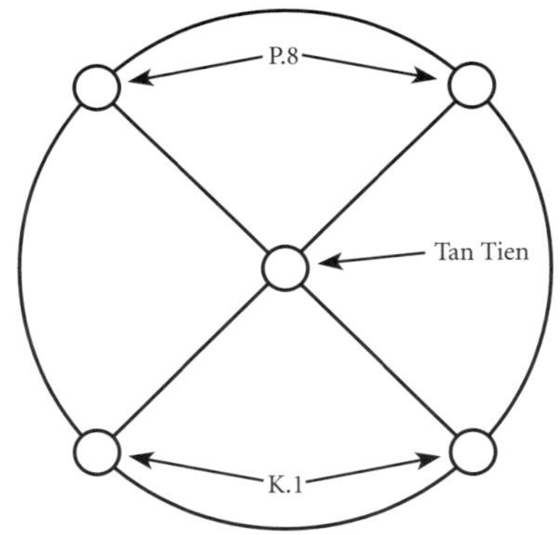

Condensing Chi Kung exploits the condensing and contracting properties of chi and its natural association with the 'element' Metal.

Firstly, fire up the chi as in Section 1, Part 3. Then the chi is extended as in Ball Breathing (*see fig.18*), in a regular front or back stance as in fig.16a and fig.16b, outward to the extremities being P.8, K.1 and GV.22 on an out or yang breath. The figure on the left is in schematic form to show the channels and is not a Chi Kung posture. Then on an in or yin breath, the thought chi is drawn into the bones of the human body by visualisation. The figure on the right is a schematic example of visualising 'conscious chi' into the skeletal structure.

Initially, it is easier to commence the visualisation process, by starting with the feet and working one's way up the body in stages, until the whole cycle can be carried out in one yin in and one yang out breath. Repeat in blocks of four.

The 'ball' above is a schematic diagram of the channels on the out yang breath.

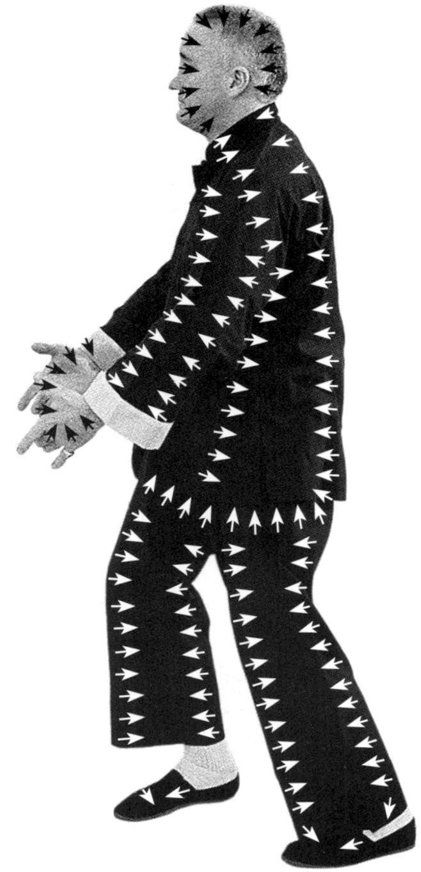

Figure 18: **Ball Breathing leading to Condensing Breath Bone Marrow Breathing.**

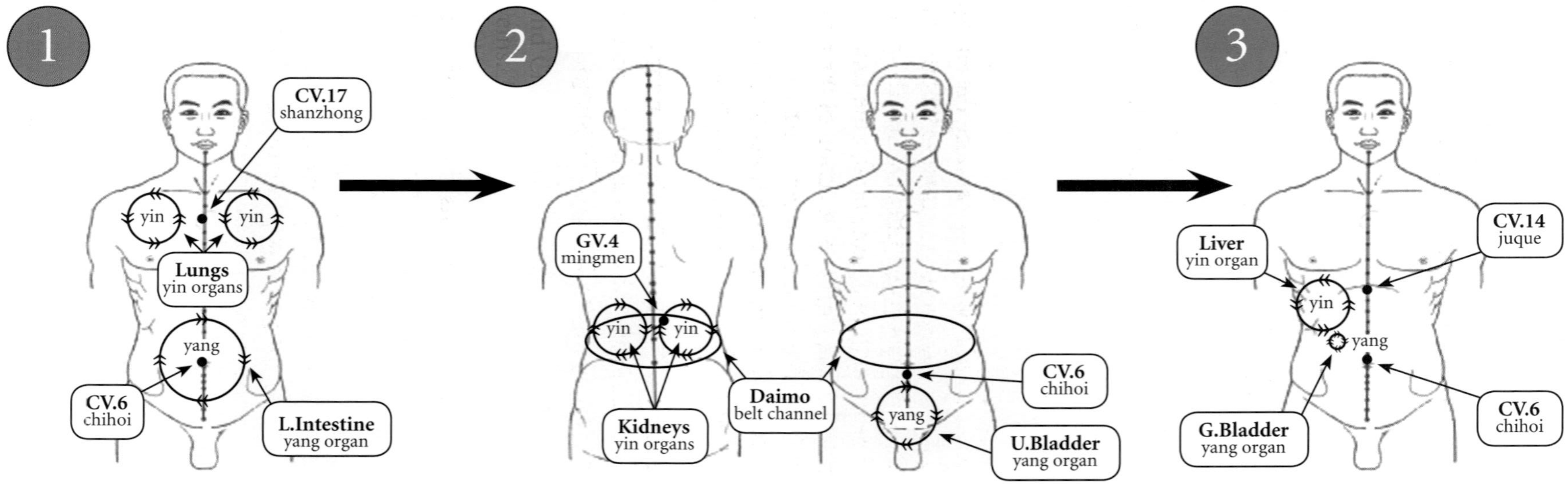

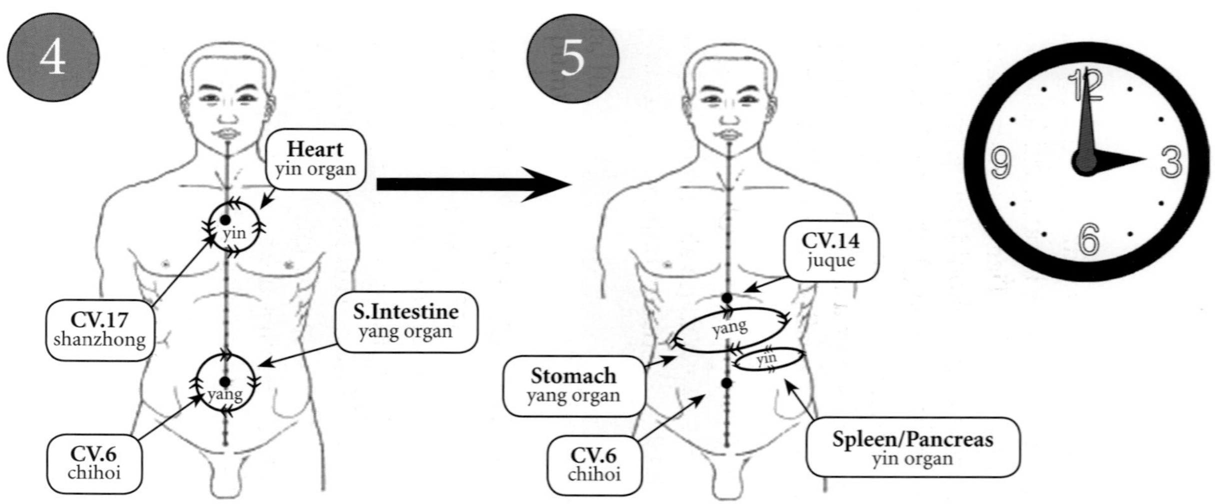

5 Element Breathing is the term which describes when chi is visualised to encircle the internal organs in a specific manner. The order is laid out in the figures 1-5 and detailed in Section 8, Part 3.

Chi has its own type of memory, so when chi is visualised in the approximate area of the required organ, the chi will naturally flow in the desired manner around the desired organ. However the chi has to be visualised in the specific spiral and direction relating to the chi of that organ.

Therefore follow the direction of the arrows which show the correct direction which relates to each organ. A yang organ requires a yang spiral, which is clockwise and the yin action for a yin organ is anti-clockwise. The direction relates to each organ in the following manner. The direction of the clockwise or anti-clockwise spiral is determined by visualising that one has a clock on the front of one's torso with the face of the clock facing outward.

Figure 19: **Five Element Breathing.**

limbs is stagnated when the body weight is evenly distributed on both feet. The arms should be held in a circular fashion as if embracing a barrel, with the fingers kept about a hands width apart, horizontal to the shoulders, the elbows and shoulders kept loose and down. The weight always held over the Yongquan (K.1) in a 70-30% bias with the toes slightly turned in, following the essentials of Central Equilibrium whenever possible.

Chi Storing

1a). After completing a set of breaths one must always store the chi at the Tan Tien, this is achieved by focusing the mind at the Chihoi (CV.6) with the hands cupped and placed as in 1) above, for about a minute or so until the sensations of energy subside. If the mind is concentrated at this point it will store the chi for later use. This can also be used to calm the chi if one has been adversely excited or stressed or to centre the chi when one is ill, as an aid to recovery. This exercise can be carried out seated, standing or lying down.

Chi Centring

1b). To assist 1a), one can imagine the chi is parked safely in this area by centring the energy in the following routine because chi follows mind intent. One needs to visualise that the chi is spiralling in the Tan Tien, about the size of a small ball that could fit easily into the palm of the hand. Women should firstly imagine chi to be turning in a neat spiral, nine times in a clockwise fashion (yang), then twelve times anticlockwise (yin). The direction of the rotations are determined by an imagined 'clock' which is laid flat on the stomach with the 'time' facing outwards. For a man it is the contrary, starting with nine yin rotations finished off by twelve yang visualised spirals. This exercise can be carried out seated, standing or lying down. (*fig.20*)

Although the principle of reverse breathing is integrated into all Chi Kungs and the Tai Chi form, it is also a stand alone method to build and stimulate chi, as well as being a precursor, acting like a choke to build up fire power before doing more advanced Chi Kungs.

Microcosmic Orbit

2). The 'micro-cosmic' orbit (*fig.16a*) is where the chi begins and ends its circuit in the Tan Tien. Firstly, the chi is thought up the Dumo meridian by way of the Huiyin (CV.1) then up along the spine, over the head on the yin, 'in breath' and on the out yang breath the chi is directed down the Renmo channel, on the anterior side of the torso back into the Tan Tien by way of the Huiyin. This should be carried out in cycles of four and not overdone to begin with. Measuring any side effects, like light headedness, changes in appetite or moods and dream activity, against the amount and frequency of the cycles. This exercise can be carried out seated, standing or lying down in blocks of four.

Macrocosmic Orbit

3). Macro cosmic breathing (*fig.16b*), is an extension of 2), where one starts by bringing chi up the spine over the head as in the micro cosmic orbit and when one exhales the chi is ideated down the Conception Vessel, continuing to descend along the middle inner part of each leg, being the central 'extra' channel of the leg known as the Yinweimo (*fig.16b*), over the inside of the ankle and terminating at the Yongquan (K.1) of both feet. The yin 'in breath' takes the chi up over the outer edge of the foot and along the outer median aspect of the legs along the 'extra' channel of the Yangweimo (*fig.16b*); then still on the 'in breath' continuing up the Dumo of the spine, ending at the top lip (GV.28), ready for the next circuit. This exercise can be carried out seated, standing or lying down in blocks of four.

Ball Breathing

4). In the 'ball breathing' (*fig.17*), one imagines that the body and limbs are the X shaped stays of an expanding and contracting sphere, the centre of the X being the Tan Tien; the front being the Chihoi and the back of the X is the Mingmen, gate of life (GV.4). One must imagine that the chi is expanding and contracting like a ball even though one is standing in the standard Chi Kung stance. To assist the process one can sink the weight slightly on the yang cycle, then raise and expand one's posture on the yin, in breath, by 10% or so. One extends the chi to the hands and feet simultaneously along the yang aspect of the X. One starts at the Tan Tien, ideating the chi along the yang side of the legs and feet, ending the out breath at the Yongquan, bubbling well (K.1), coinciding with chi ascending up the Dumo, then outward to the arms at the Shenzu (GV.12) continuing along the yang sides of the arms over the hands and middle fingers, finishing at the Laogong, the palace of hard work (P.8) in the centre of the palms. The chi is then withdrawn along the yin aspects of the legs and arms back to the Tan Tien for further rounds. To conclude simply, during the yang outward breath, the chi follows the Dumo then the meridians of the Triple Heater of the arms and the 'extra' meridian of the median line of the leg Yangweimo. On the yin breath the chi is withdrawn along the Pericardium channel of the arm and hand, and the 'extra' meridian of the Yinweimo being the midline channel on the yin side of the leg, ending by flowing up the Conception Vessel back to the Chihoi, where the chi is returned to the Tan Tien for storage or further cycles. This exercise can be carried out seated or standing in blocks of four.

Condensing Breath

5). The Condensing Breath (*fig.18*), is where after firing up the chi one does a yang 'ball' breath, as in 4), then on the yin in breath the chi is ideated into the very bone structures by visualisation. One has to imagine the chi surrounding the skeletal structure as a circular field of energy which is contracting and condensing evenly inwards. When one becomes more proficient one can train the chi to penetrate the hollows of every bone however small. To begin with, it is easier to imagine this process in stages, by starting the condensing procedure in the bones of the feet, up into the legs, the pelvis, ribs, spine, arms, hands and the skull and so forth. Eventually one will be able to condense the chi inwards to the whole skeleton in one yin action. It is not too important to have a precise knowledge of anatomy. Bone is fairly obviously situated and chi 'knows' the body and will be able to home in on an ideated target. This Chi Kung strengthens the bones, fortifies the marrow and acts like a fuel cell, storing chi. It was also used to temper the limbs for martial practice and can be integrated in Fa Jing techniques assisting to fire chi outwards. As the chi becomes more assimilated with 'mind intent', the wavelength is shortened by the will from a long wave to a short wave just like a radio signal, making the chi sharper and more concentrated. This exercise can be carried out seated, standing or lying down in blocks of four. Stem cells are stored in the marrow, as well as many facets of the blood and immune function. The condensing breath can store chi in the bone like a rechargeable battery as well as stimulating the various cells in the marrow.

Heaven and Earth Breath

6). Heaven and Earth Breathing is best carried out early morning in a natural comfortable place. One starts with reverse breathing and then on the in breath one imagines that the 'chi' of Heaven and the Earth is drawn in simultaneously. The upper Heaven chi is visualised as passing down through the Baihui (GV.20), descending the spine along to the end of the Renmo then through the Huiyin (CV.1) up to the Tan Tien. Simultaneously Earth chi is drawn up by way of the Laogong (K.1) points of both feet, along the yin aspect of the legs and the Conception Vessel of the body into the Tan Tien. Both Heaven and Earth chi meeting at the Tan Tien at the same time. One can use the ball breathing and or condensing Chi Kung to accompany and enhance chi assimilation. A martial extension of Heaven and Earth Chi Kung was adapted to greatly increase the root of stances by ideating the chi into the ground through the feet to an imagined depth of about six inches on the out breath or technique and think up on the yin in breath and so forth. Repeat in cycles of four which can be mixed and matched with 1), 2), 3), 4) & 5). Science is now able to measure the various forces that travel across space such as neutrinos etc. as well as gravity passing through material structures including human beings and the Earth itself. The Taoist Masters had sensed these forces, recognising the downward force as the chi of Heaven being a contracting yang chi and the upward yin energy, expanding as the chi of the Earth returning into space.

Twelve Meridians Breathing

7). Meridian Breathing is commenced after the chi is fanned, by reverse breathing. One will need to obtain a fairly comprehensive acupuncture chart to carry out this Chi Kung where the meridians are clearly defined. As usual one begins with 1) then on a yin breath one brings the chi up the Conception Vessel directing the chi to the beginning of both lung meridians at the hollows next to the shoulders at (Lu.1), Zhonfu. The first of twelve breaths is a yang out breath where the chi is envisaged to travel down the lung channel. Then the chi is taken around the body simulating the course of energy from the twenty-four hour cycle of chi as it passes through the twelve meridians; terminating at the end of the liver channel in the chest; where, still on the last in breath, the chi is taken up through the Conception Vessel, into the Governing Vessel, up through the eyes, over the Baihui (GV.20) down the spine, passing through the Huiyin (CV.1) and finishing in the Conception Vessel at the Chihoi (CV.6), finally returning the chi to the Tan Tien.

The chi is directed in this order through the channels starting with the:-

Lung Channel* (yang, out breath) - to the ***Large Intestine Channel* (yin, in breath) to the,
****Stomach Channel*** (yang breath) - to the ***Spleen/Pancreas Channel*** (yin breath) to the,
****Heart Channel*** (yang breath) - to the ***Small Intestine Channel*** (yin breath) to the,

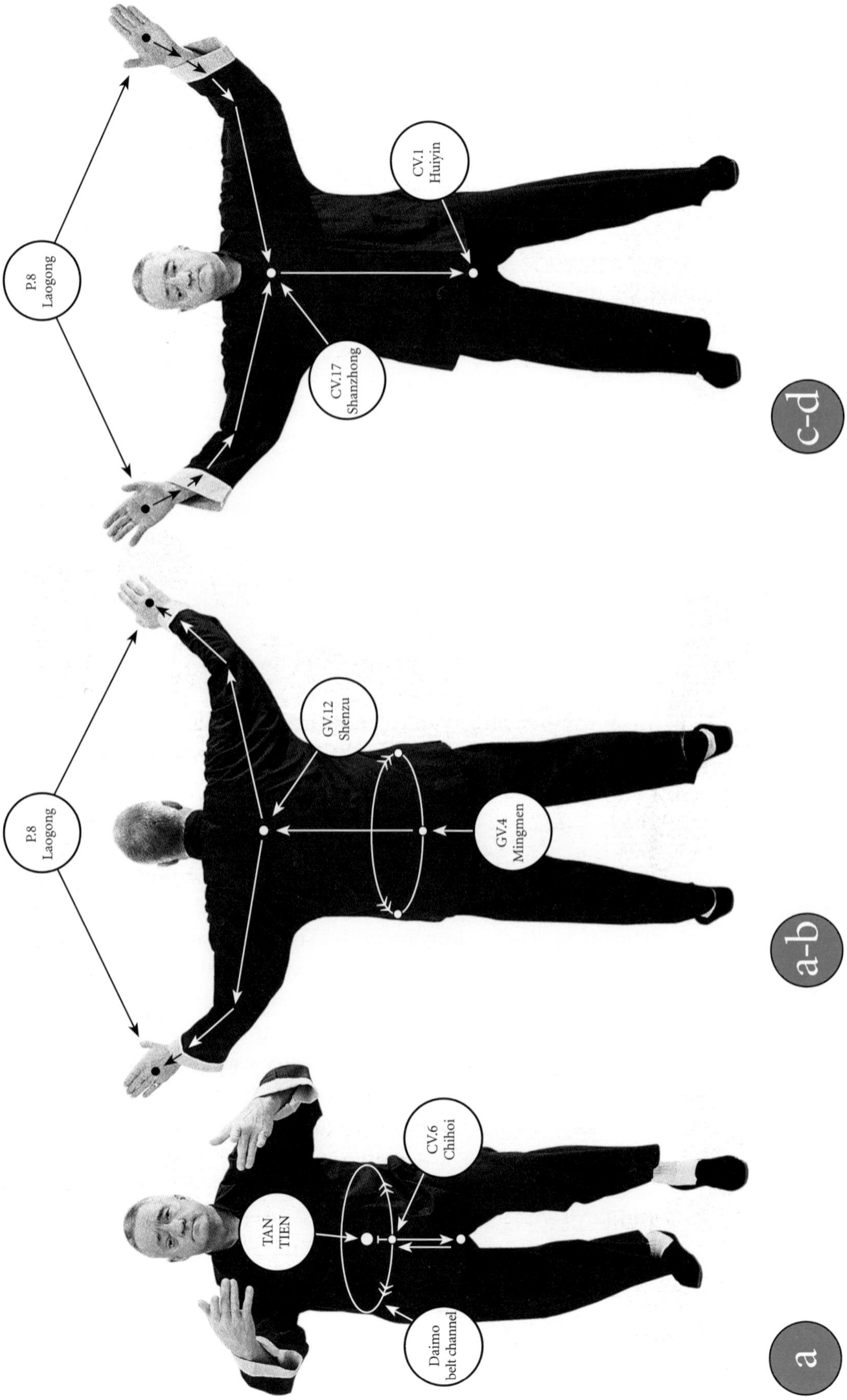

Figure 20a: **Eight Trigram Breathing.**

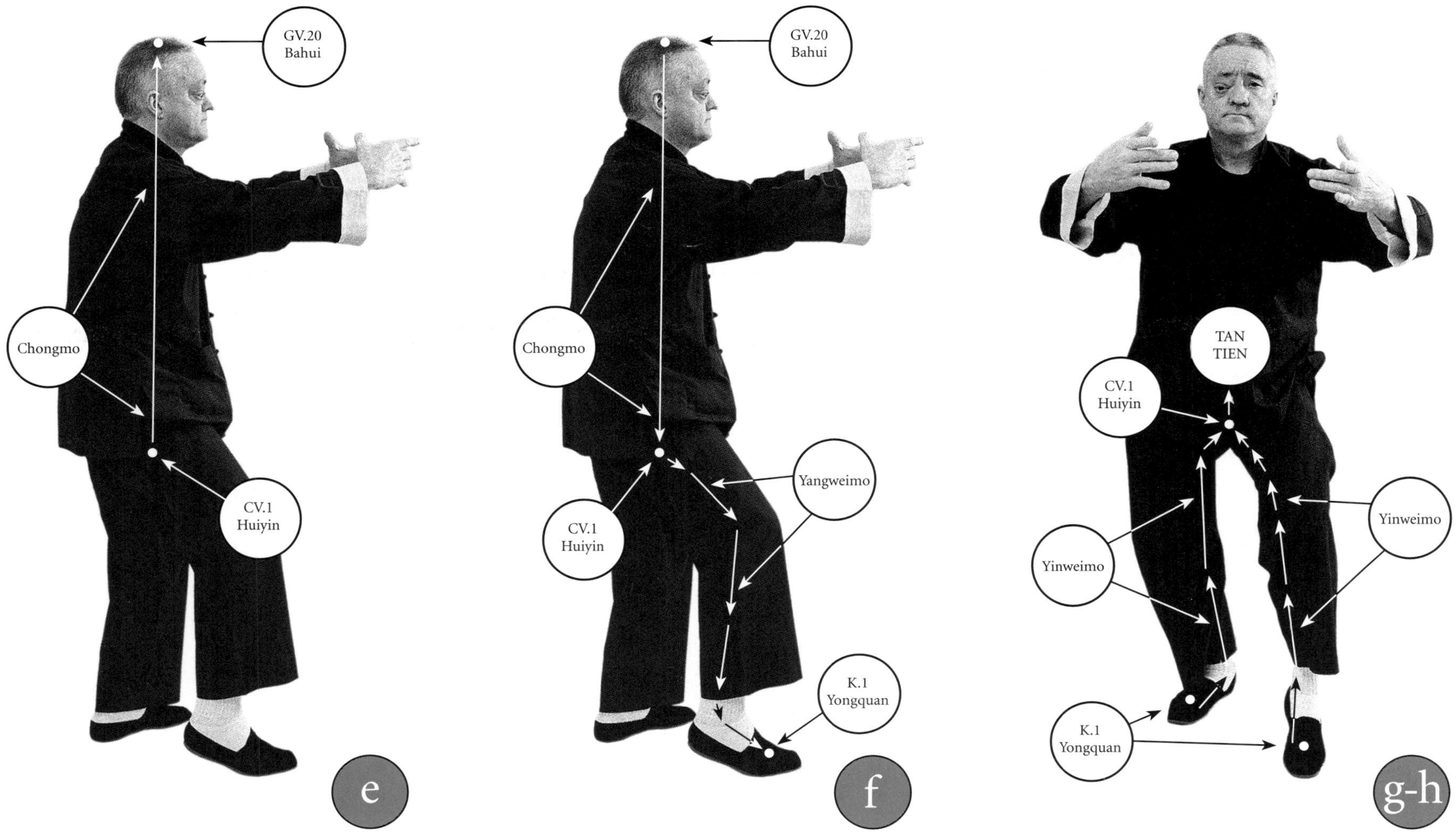

Figure 20b: **BaQua Breathing** - Please refer to Section 9, Part 3 where the visualisation process of the 8 trigram breathing is described in detail. This Chi Kung should be carried out in a posture as in (**a**) - (**g**) - (**h**). The other postures are shown schematically in order to show where the chi is to be focussed. This Chi Kung can be carried out in a front or back stance (fig. 15). The lettering, laid out in figures 20a and 20b, follows the order in Section 9, Part 3. So, figure (**a**) = 9a and (**a-b**) = 9a and 9b, finishing with (**g-h**), being 9g and 9h and so forth.

Urinary Bladder Channel* (yang breath) - to the ***Kidney Channel* (yin breath) to the,
Pericardium Channel* (yang breath) - to the ***Triple Heater Channel* (yin breath) to the,
Gall Bladder Channel* (yang breath) - to the ***Liver Channel* (yin breath), on the final yin breath the chi is drawn up the ***Renmo Channel***, through the ***Dumo Channel*** then back up the ***Renmo*** into the ***Tan Tien*** in one step.

It is advisable to do once a day only, preferably A.M. and no more than one block of four to begin with. This exercise can be carried out seated, standing or lying down.

Five Element Breathing

8). The Five Element Internal Organ Breathing (*fig.19*). After a firing and build up of chi in the Tan Tien:

**Lung* - The first yin breath takes the chi up the Conception Vessel to the lung area, to the sternum, acupoint Shanzhong (CV.17) where one imagines the chi to bifurcate over each lung and still on this in breath one visualises for the rest of the yin breath, two anti-clockwise spirals (the yin/yang direction of the circling as in 1b).

**Large Intestine* - The next out breath takes the chi down the Conception Vessel to acupoint Chihoi (CV.6) and still on the out breath the chi is circled in a yang clockwise spiral around the outer rim of the abdominal cavity where the Large Intestine is situated.

**Kidney* - During the next in yin spiral and breath, the chi is drawn around the Daimo, the belt channel which runs around the waist from the Chihoi (CV.6) to the Mingmen gate (GV.4) where the chi is bifurcated in two yin spirals around each kidney,

**Bladder* - after which the yang out breath retraces the belt channel to the Chihoi (CV.6) where the chi is yang spiralled over the urinary bladder in the lower abdominal cavity behind the pubic bone.

**Liver* - Next the chi is drawn up the Conception Vessel to acupoint Juque (CV.14) and yin chi is spiralled over the liver on the in breath around the lower right ribcage,

**Gall Bladder* - followed by a yang breath with a small spiral (1 inch in diameter) around the gall bladder which is situated midway on the underside of the left lobe of the liver, about half way along the line of the lowest right rib.

**Heart* - Next the chi is drawn along the Conception Vessel to the Shanzhong (CV.17) and yin circled, the size of one's fist, around the heart which lies slightly to the left of this acupoint.

**Small Intestine* - The out breath takes the chi down to the Chihoi (CV.6) where a smallish yang cycle, about the width of one's palm, is carried out around the small intestine.

**Spleen/Pancreas* - The final yin breath taking the chi up the Conception Vessel to the Juque

(CV.14) and yin spiralled about the spleen/pancreas which is approximately under and one hand size to the left of Juque (CV.14) under the left ribcage finally,

**Stomach* - leading to the last yang breath and cycled over the stomach.

As with 7) it should only be done in one block of four once a day AM. This exercise can be carried out seated, standing or lying down. In this order:-

***Metal - Lung** (yin, in breath and spiral) to ***Large Intestine** (yang, out breath and spiral) to,
***Water - Kidneys** (yin breath and spiral) to ***Bladder** (yang breath and spiral) to,
***Wood - Liver** (yin breath and spiral) to ***Gallbladder** (yang breath and spiral) to,
***Fire - Heart** (yin breath and spiral) to ***Small Intestine** (yang breath and spiral) to,
***Earth - Spleen/Pancreas** (yin breath and spiral) to ***Stomach** (yang breath and spiral).

Eight Trigram Breathing

9). Eight Trigram Breathing (*figs.20a/20b*) is so called because it takes chi around the body in such a way as it stimulates all the chi channels especially the eight extra meridians which are connected to the eight trigrams. The chi is fired up in the Tan Tien by reverse breathing then:-

a) on an in breath it is drawn to the Chihoi (CV.6) around the Daimo, belt channel to the Mingmen (GV.4) up along the Governing Vessel to the mid-point between the shoulder blades, Shenzhu (GV.12),

b) then on the out breath the chi is directed from the Shenzhu (GV.12), in a straight line down the outside yang aspect of the arms and hands to the Laogong (P.8),

c) the chi is withdrawn on a yin breath on the yin side of the arms to the Shanzhong (CV.17) on the sternum,

d) the next out breath takes the energy down the Conception Vessel to the Huiyin (CV.1),

e) the chi is drawn up on the yin breath along the Chongmo, one of the 'extra' channels that runs in a straight line up the front of the body linking the Huiyin (CV.1) with the Baihui (GV.20) directly,

f) the following breath is a yang expiration sending the chi down along the Chongmo through the Huiyin (CV.6) then on and down the Yangweimo of the outer median aspect of each leg to the Yongquan (K.1) of both feet.

g) the yin breath brings the chi back up the inner median sides of the legs, the Yinweimo, through the Huiyin (CV.1) and the first part of the Chongmo to the Tan Tien.

h) On the eighth and final yang breath, one relaxes the mind and focuses the energy back at the Tan Tien.

As with the micro-cosmic orbit 2) this breathing exercise, which is more dynamic, must be gauged against any unusual effects relating to the amount of practice. This Chi Kung links the upper and lower parts of the mind and body. Do only once a day in blocks of four in the morning AM. This exercise can be carried out seated, standing or lying down.

Fa Ching - Chi Kung

10). To obtain focused healing chi or martial chi one has to do at least one hour of Chi Kung and or several intrinsic Tai Chi forms each day. The Chi Kungs should be a mix and match of all the afore mentioned with an emphasis on 1), 2), 3), 4, 5) & 6). When chi is becoming very clear and one is able to move it at will, possibly after two to three years of consistent training, one can start taking postures from the Tai Chi repertoire, (*Refer* to my book ***Tai Chi Chuan and The Code of Life***) and direct chi into the different parts of the hand and fingers in order to be able to focus the internal energy to heal others. The dark side of this technique was used in Tai Chi's martial practices.

For example, a left style 'Push' stance from 'Grasp Bird's Tail' (*Refer* to my book ***Tai Chi Chuan and The Code of Life***) with the weight being mainly over the left leg, the essence of this stance being to form an internal chi spiral of energy, a connected Chan Shu Jian, from the left foot to the right palm. The posture is adopted, Chi Kung style, and after fanning the fire, one ideates most of the chi into the base of the palm. This will induce an 'inner' anti-clockwise spiral of Chan Shu Jian chi, joining the Yongquan (K.1) of the left foot around the left leg, across the body down the arm into the right palm at the Laogong, (P.8). As well as focusing chi into the palm, making it ready for healing transmission, it will also stimulate the Fire chi of the practitioner.

Thus all the postures of the Original Yang Style energise and balance the chi of specific channels, in this case the organs of circulation and metabolism. My Tai Chi teacher, Master Chu told me a story from his adopted father, Yang Shou Chung, how the Yang family would joke and laugh amongst themselves, if they ever became embroiled in a fight, however serious, because not only would they polish their martial skills but also energise their meridians, keeping them healthier.

As in every stance and technique of the 'Original Yang Style Chi Kung, a 'thought chi' memory will be built up and stored. This retains the chi intention of that posture, coupled with the inner meanings and techniques of the Classic Thirteen Postures of Tai Chi.

This will allow a build up of internal energy which can be used for healing, art, reinforce career potential, martial practices as well as to create and maintain one's health.

PART FOUR

Conclusion

To conclude, be as natural as possible, but consciously. That is, follow the Universal Principle expounded in this book relating it to your own psyche and experience.

I used the yin yang nomenclature, albeit Chinese in origin, as a vehicle to explain this simple yet dynamic law. Yin and yang although sometimes derided or misunderstood is now global terminology. The yin yang symbol can be seen on surf boards, temples, all over the internet and body tattoos, to name but a few examples.

These opposite antagonistic properties have been recognised in all cultures, as simply the feminine and masculine or deified like Shiva and Shakti in the Hindu culture. Heraclitus in ancient Greece c. 500 BC noted that the world was in a state of constant change between opposites. Isaac Newton realised that *"every action has its equal and opposite reaction"*. The I Ching c. 2600 B.C. declares that the *"only constant is change"*. Besides many more such as Mother Earth, Father Sky, Jaweh and Sophia, Mohamed and Fatima, Jesus as sponsus and church as sponsa, conscious and unconscious and so forth. Western science tabulates these laws in the atom as the proton's positive charge and the electron's negative charge, last but not least the plus and minus attributes in the binary code that makes up the double strand of the helix of DNA.

Once understood it can be applied to any and all factors of life, whether physical or psychical. It is useful, as it is an empirical method of looking at both the inner and outer worlds. If more people apply this Universal Principle or law, our lonely yet sacred planet and its peoples and environment stand a better chance.

Bibliography

_____. *Barefoot Doctor's Manual.* Prepared by the Revolutionary Health Committee of Hunan Province. Routledge Kegan Paul London 1997.

Bartram, Thomas. *Bartram's Encyclopedia of Herbal Medicine.* Robinson. London 1995.

_____. *Britannica CD 98.* Encylopaedia Britannica Inc. Chicago 1998.

Chang, Dr. Stephen. *The Complete Book of Acupuncture.* Celestial Arts. Berkeley 1976.

——— *The Tao of Sexology—The Book of Wisdom.* Tao Publishing. San Francisco 1988.

Connelly, Diane. *Traditional Acupuncture—The Law of the Five Elements.* Center for Traditional Acupuncture Inc. Maryland 1979.

Eisenberg, M.D., David. *Encounters with Qi.* Norton & Co. Ltd. New York 1995.

_____. *Encylopaedia Britannica.* Encylopaedia Britannica Inc. Chicago 1996.

Huang, Wen Shan. *Fundamentals of Tai Chi Chuan.* South Sky Book Co. Hong Kong/ Seattle 1982.

_____. *I Ching.* Translated by Richard Wilhelm. Routledge Kegan Paul. London 1989.

Jing, Chen. *Anatomical Atlas of Chinese Acupuncture.* Shandong Science & Technology Press. Jinan 1982.

Jung, C. G. *Collected Works of C. G. Jung.* Routledge Kegan Paul. London 1985.

Kenyon, Julian. *Modern Acupuncture Techniques.* Thorsons. Wellingborough, UK, 1982.

Ki Sun. *The Cannon of Acupuncture.* Yuin University Press. Los Angeles 1985.

Kushi, Michio. *How to See Your Health Book of Oriental Diagnosis.* Japan Publications Inc. Tokyo 1980.

Lau, D. C. *Lao Tzu—Tao Te Ching.* Penguin Books. London 1976.

Muramoto, Naboru. Healing Ourselves. Swan House Publishing. London 1975.

Needham, Joseph. Science & Civilisation in China. Cambridge Press. Cambridge 1976.

_____. *Oxford Concise Medical Dictionary.* Oxford University Press. Oxford/New York 1996.

_____. *Oxford Interactive Encyclopedia (CD).* The Learning Company. Oxford 1997.

Ping, Dr. Wu Wei. *Chinese Acupuncture.* Health Science Press. Wellingborough, UK, 1974.

Quan, Lui Bing. *Optimum Time of Acupuncture.* Shandong Science & Technology Press. Jinan 1988.

Veith, Ilza. *Yellow Emperor's Classic of Internal Medicine.* University of California Press. Los Angeles 1972.

Wile, Douglas. *Yang Family Secret Transmissions.* Sweet Chi Press. New York 1983.

Wiseman, Ellis. *Fundamentals of Chinese Medicine.* Paradigm Publications. Brooklin, Mass, 1985.

_____. *"The Wonders of Qigong."* China Sports Magazine. Wayfarer Publications. Los Angeles 1972.

Yongsheng, Bi. *Chinese Qigong—Outgoing Qi Therapy.* Shandong Science & Technology Press. Jinan 1992.

Yongsheng, Bi, and Sun Hua, Guo Yi, Cao Zhenhua, Zhang Mingqin, Zhang Bohua. *Chinese Qigong.* Shanghai College of Traditional Medicine. Shanghai 1990.

Index

O

P

Q

R

S

T

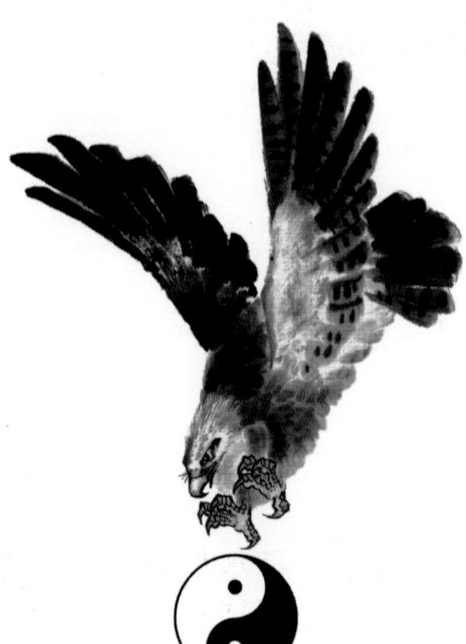

Taoist Group Publishers
www.taichi-horwood.com